When Was Arts in Health?

Frances Williams

When Was Arts in Health?

A History of the Present

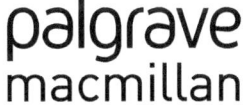

Frances Williams
Glyndwr University
Wrexham, UK

ISBN 978-981-19-3616-6   ISBN 978-981-19-3617-3   (eBook)
https://doi.org/10.1007/978-981-19-3617-3

This Palgrave Macmillan imprint is published by the registered company Springer Nature Singapore Pte Ltd.
The registered company address is: 152 Beach Road, #21-01/04 Gateway East, Singapore 189721, Singapore

For my late parents, Mr Edmund and Dr Margaret Williams

Acknowledgements

This book was written between summer 2021 and spring 2022, during the ongoing pandemic, following the completion of my PhD in late 2019. My viva was conducted over Zoom, a novel form of communication at that time, in the week when the national lockdown began in March 2020. These events have informed the writing of this book in many ways, extending points made in my original thesis, while rendering others obsolete. I have tried to develop arguments in step with rapidly unfolding events. I finished writing a draft in spring 2022, just as the government published its White Paper on 'levelling-up', a government still led at this time by Boris Johnson despite ongoing calls for his resignation. Liz Truss had replaced Johnson at the book's proofing stage in Autumn 2022 and, as I write, political chaos ensues sending markets into turmoil.

I would like to thank those who held enough faith in my work to publish it over this tragic, uncertain period: Victoria Hume (creative health & Wellbeing Alliance), Angela Rogers (Wales Arts, Health and Well-being Network); Will Davies (Political Economy Research Centre), Stephen Pritchard and Stephen Clift (Frontiers), Tehseen Noorani (Polyphony), Janina Kehr and Fanny Chabrol (Somatosphere), Lindsey Colborne and all the crew (Utopias Bach) and Emily Trahair (Planet).

I was also supported by my colleagues at Glyndwr University (Sue Liggett, Anthony Jackson) and all the MA staff and students there who taught me valuable life lessons. Thanks to all those in the Critical Arts and Health Network who remain an ongoing source of support and inspiration (Becky Shaw, Anthony Schrag and Sarah Smizz). Further thanks to my friend Dr Wanda Zyborska for encouragements throughout. And the work of the two editors at Palgrave who pushed the book in and out of production (Joshua Pitt, Marion Duval).

Enormous thanks go to my PhD Supervisor, Dr Clive Parkinson, and Director of Studies, Professor Amanda Ravetz. Without Clive's encouragement to apply for a doctoral scholarship at Manchester Metropolitan University in 2015, none of this work would have been possible. His work upholds so much of the radical tradition on which the Arts for Health was first established in the city of Manchester. This book relies entirely on all the generosities listed above. Lastly, thanks to my family. To Rachel who subsidised time lost to the writing of this book with patience and good humour. I dedicate it finally to my late parents, whose lives were so shaped by their respective birth place, now also resting place: The Rhondda Valley.

CONTENTS

LIST OF FIGURES

CHAPTER 1

Who Calls Time?

Let's begin with two narratives that oddly collide in time, one of tragic closure, the other cast as hopeful opening. March 2020 marked the month when the UK government decided to impose the first ever national lockdown in response to the spread of a new corona virus.[1] At this early point in the global pandemic, COVID-19 had claimed around a thousand lives in this country. When the UK's Chief Medical Officer warned that a death toll of 20,000 would represent a "good result" should a national lockdown be implemented, this move was reluctantly conceded by the Prime Minister, Boris Johnson. In the same month, a new UK institution was born: The National Centre for creative health (NCCH). Though representing minor news by comparison, the aim set out by this new body was nevertheless an ambitious one. The NCCH would "mainstream" arts interventions in healthcare, playing "a pivotal role" in "promoting collaboration to enable creative health to become integral to health and social care systems".[2] But what is 'creative health' and why was a new national centre needed to advance it so? Why might its launch, at this most anxious point in time, mark an "exciting" and "very important moment"?

CREATIVE HEALTH

The broader concept of creative health had been so-named three years earlier by an All Party Parliamentary Group (APPG). A dedicated inquiry, begun in 2014, culminated in a 2017 report titled *creative health: the*

© The Author(s), under exclusive license to Springer Nature Singapore Pte Ltd. 2023
F. Williams, *When Was Arts in Health?*,
https://doi.org/10.1007/978-981-19-3617-3_1

Arts for Health and Wellbeing.[3] It included a plethora of case studies which aimed to evidence how art and culture could support mental and physical health. Research findings were squarely aimed at the UK government led, at this earlier time, by Teresa May.[4] In her first speech as Prime Minister, May had referred to the "burning injustice" of health inequalities across UK regions, one which saw people "born poor… die on average nine years earlier than others" (May, 2017: 1). She had insisted that the UK's "precious Union" was a bond not only between its constituent "home nations", but a union forged between individual citizens "wherever we're from" (ibid, p. 1).

Her words appeared to augur well for this APPG group given that their 2017 report was underpinned by epidemiological research into the 'causes of the causes' of ill-health, those which could evidence widening health inequalities (Marmot & Wilkinson, 1996; Marmot, 2010; Marmot, 2015).[5] The 'social determinants of health' (SDOH) were invoked as a way of understanding how good health could be promoted across all regions and nations of the UK. The World Health Organisation's (WHO) definition of SDOH was advanced as a key theory underpinning the adoption of creative health: "The conditions in which people are born, grow, work, live, and age, and the wider set of forces and systems shaping the conditions of daily life" (APPGAHW, 2017: 10).

Art and culture, the report went further in suggesting, can be seen as an "essential vaccine" in the wider "immunization package" of decent living conditions shown to protect individual and collective health (ibid, p. 30).[6] The health benefits of participation in arts and culture were set over the life course. Chapters were dedicated to creative projects aimed at those in their early years, adolescence, working years and old age. 'Culture' was defined broadly, not merely involving the placement of paintings on hospital (or gallery) walls, but encompassing ordinary everyday activities, grassroot "community cultural festivals, fairs" (Davies et al., 2012). It was aimed squarely at "people who have to make policy decisions, funding decisions and clinical decisions", as these were considered best placed to "unlock change" (ibid, p. 7).

The establishment of the NCCH was one of the report's ten recommendations, all of which were informed by directions already set in motion by NHS managers and cultural sector leaders. Many were to be enacted at a local, as much as national, level. Recommendation four, for example, demanded that "arts and cultural organizations are involved in the delivery of health and wellbeing at regional and local level" (APPGAHW, 2017: 15).

While recommendation five urged that the public body responsible for supporting the arts in England, Arts Council England (ACE), "make health and wellbeing outcomes integral to their work", identifying "health and wellbeing as a priority in its 10-year strategy" (APPGAHW: 150).

By way of such emphasis, local arts organisations funded by ACE would be encouraged to orientate their participatory programmes explicitly towards health outcomes. This was an integration proposed despite reservations having been raised by many researchers in preceding years about the illusionary, even "coerced" nature of participation deployed in gallery and museum settings (Lynch & Alberti, 2010; Lynch, 2013; Marstine, 2011; Sandell & Nightingale, 2012). One arts consultancy group noted, for example, how duties of accountability were dangerously skewed to government agendas over needs identified by local communities themselves (Holden et al., 2014). Governance of local arts bodies, they warned, should "reflect community" and not "mistake public funding as a proxy for public engagement" (ibid, p. 2).[7]

Similar concerns were raised around new developments in healthcare. Restructurings of the NHS would be modelled on regional footprints through the introduction of Sustainability and Transformation Plans (STPs). The APPGAHW report recommendation that arts organisations be "involved in the delivery of health and well-being at a local level" was advocated without reference to health workers and researchers who believed that STPs constituted "a recipe for a chronically under-resourced, chaotic and scandal-prone NHS" (Lister, 2017: 15). STPs, their opponents argued, would adversely impact patient care through the adoption of US style models of "accountable care" (El Gingihy, 2017; Lister et al., 2015; Lister, 2017).[8] "Accountability to accountants and not to patient's clinical needs" (Land, 2018).

Across both the arts and health sectors then, public participation, engagement and accountability were identified as weak, easily by-passed or co-opted, "vulnerable to political agendas" (Lynch, 2013: 13). Recommendation eight in the report centred on learning. It urged UK universities to set up courses that were "dedicated to the contribution of the arts to health and wellbeing" (APPGAHW, 2017: 155). These modules would sit between the Arts and Sciences, part of a broader trend to foster interdisciplinary exchange. Yet even here, the notion of interdisciplinarity had been identified as in need of "re-thinking" due to logics which "obviate inequality" across "territories" brought into being in this way (Fitzgerald & Callard, 2015: 86).

Many tensions then, borne of unequal relationships—between publicly funded institutions and their publics, systems of knowledge and power—ran as potential complication to the report's ten recommendations. Rather than broach these points, recommendations flowed in the direction of strategies already set by in place by leaders in the arts, health and education sectors. Their implementation would represent more of an endorsement of existing power structures and strategy than mount any challenge to them. Yet the creation of the new NCCH was heralded by way of radical change, rather than continuity by APPG Chair, Lord Howarth. He presented this moment in March 2020 as an "opportunity to make a difference", one informed by the belief that:

> active engagement with the arts and culture – whether through our own creative practice or through our enjoyment of the creative practice of others – is beneficial for the wellbeing and health of all of us (Howarth, 2020)

This was an affirmation made without any qualification of who "others" might be or how they might, or might not, constitute "all of us". Nor was any further detail provided on what "engagement" with culture might involve, beyond it being "active". In fact, the only negative reference to any *specific* culture in the whole of the APPGAHW report is made in relation to "the culture of healthcare" in the NHS as this "tends too much towards the technical-industrial and bureaucratic" (APPGAHW, 2017: 6). This was the only hint of critique in an advocacy document delayed to fit the political moment of opportunity presented in 2017—one which saw the narrow defeat of a Labour Party led by Jeremy Corbyn by Teresa May.

The announcement of the launch of the NCCH, then, was not informed by any clear distinction between what creative health agenda might be designed to fight against relative to what it might be fighting *for*. The role of the NCCH was not to encourage speculation on these finer points, as its sister body might, the creative health and Well-Being Alliance (CHWA). This had been simultaneously created as a new membership body in England, one comprising over 6000 individuals and groups. Only the NCCH would take on the role of providing a "strategic overview" across all tiers of UK government, working "independently" but "closely with governments" based across the four nations—it was clarified by Howarth from his crossbench seat in the House of Lords.[9] The NCCH was, and remains, an unlocated virtual entity.

HEALTH CRISIS, CULTURE WAR

The NCCH was unveiled ahead of a year of global pandemic which saw diverse social movements demand creative health by urgent, alternate means. In June 2020, Black Lives Matter (BLM) protests sprang-up in the United States of America (USA) in response to the murder of George Floyd by a State Police Officer. As part of calls for justice in relation to this case, protestors further challenged the continuing presence of public statues erected in memory of confederate war heroes—seen as the cultural emblems of a resurgent white supremacism, tacitly endorsed by President Trump since there were "very fine people on both sides".[10]

Protestors objected to colonial statues continuing public presence in the UK too. In June 2020, in the regional city of Bristol, the statue of slave merchant Edward Colston was joyfully toppled by residents who consigned it to the harbour's depths (Fig. 1.1). They did so to make 'space to breathe' a placard asserted, referencing Floyd's last words ("I can't breathe"). Direct action was informed by discourses which sought to re-create public spaces that might expose and combat racism, its cultural roots, expression and symbolisms. "When a statue falls, it opens a possible space of resignification in power's dense and saturated landscape… It is necessary to make room for living bodies", one art critic drew the link (Preciada, 2020: 1). In former British territories across the globe, statues erected to British monarchs would also be pulled down as part of protests mounted against colonial crimes committed in the past, compounded in the present.[11]

Global action took place in the UK, as it did in the USA, as Black and Asian communities disproportionately suffered the deadly impacts of COVID-19. Mortality rates were unevenly distributed across populations and place, revealing and deepening existing health inequalities. This was evidenced though data collected across UK regions and cities, a trend detected at all scales, including neighbourhood and street level. Contrary to the assertion made in the APPGAHW report, the NHS did not prove bureaucratically cumbersome in the face of this unprecedented public health crisis. Rather, the NHS proved itself efficient in the delivery of vaccines.[12] This contrasted with the performance of private companies charged by the Health Secretary with the task of running the 'test and trace' system, which proved wasteful by comparison (as a public Inquiry would later attest, (see note 12).

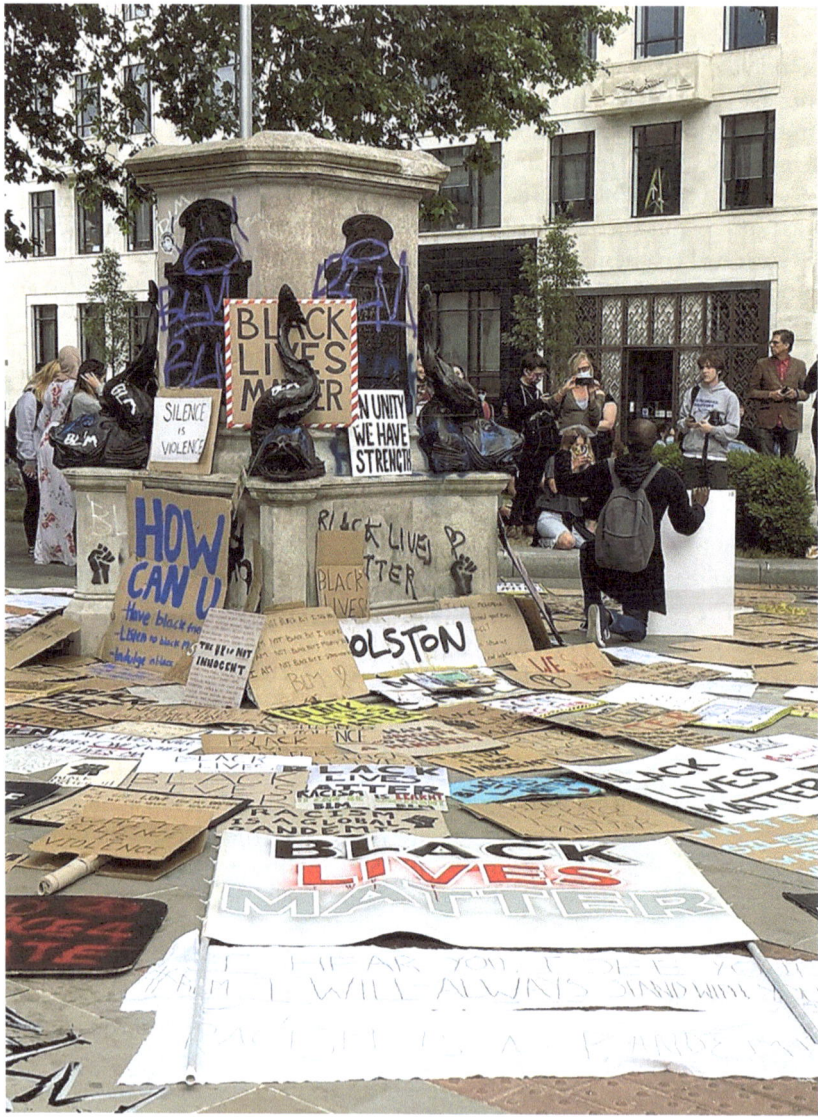

Fig. 1.1 The empty pedestal of the statue of Edward Colston in Bristol, the day after protesters toppled the statue of the slave trader and rolled it into the harbour

Simultaneously, 'culture wars' were stoked by both the UK and USA governments. Their representatives deployed motifs of foreign threat to mount appeals to nationalist sentiment over those of international cooperation. War histories allowed novel "covid nationalisms" to be staged (Davies, 2020), including fly-pasts by a Spitfire plane marked-up with 'thanks' to the NHS (a revisionist nostalgia, since the NHS was created *after* the war). The Secretary of State for Culture and Sport warned arts institutions and museums not to act on community calls to take down public statues, threatening to withdraw public funding if they did. "We won't allow Britain's history to be cancelled" (Dowden, 2021). It was observed that this prohibition was a substitution: "an attempt to obscure tackling memorials of anti-Black violence by pretending it's not human lives and bodies that are at risk but stone statues" (Hicks, 2021). A policy of 'retain and explain' was imposed on all public cultural bodies in England, demanding they prioritise this approach over the wishes of any local community.[13]

Fast forward to June 2021. Fifteen months on from the launch of the NCCH and nearly 130,000 UK citizens have died as a result of contracting the COVID-19 virus. At an International Conference on Arts, Health and Well-being hosted by CHWA, delegates spoke of the themes of "power, inequality and sustainability". Not much had changed in the tone or content of a keynote speech, titled *Gaining Ground*, delivered online by Lord Howarth. Over the last year, the movement had advanced to a "drum beat that grows more powerful" as a result of the pandemic. The "misery of covid" provided a "grim backcloth" against which the adoption of the creative health agenda was foregrounded as a bright hope. The "creative health movement" Howarth asserted:

> ...is part of a wider movement which demands justice - health justice, racial justice, social justice and climate justice. The power structures that perpetuate such injustices are not to be tolerated. Ultimately the greatest power is the power of ideas and no obstacle can withstand the power of an idea whose time has come.

The dissonant narratives recounted above open this book in order to make the case for more scrutiny of the creative health agenda—its rationale, application, value and timeliness. This book will explore the preconditions that have allowed this new descriptor to come into being, superseding the field's former iteration as 'Arts in Health' or 'Arts for Health'. I will query and problematise the promotion of the concept of creative health as advanced by the NCCH, a national body which claims to be driven by the needs and views of those belonging to a grassroots social movement. Rather, the extent to which the creative health agenda aligns with a regressive neoliberal agenda will be explored. Could it represent a set of demands that have been selectively (mis)applied? Could the longer push for Arts in Health be one that is congruent with the rise of neoliberal modes of governance? Some voices within the field suggest it might, with the arts more broadly cast as "the perfect foil for the vengeful ideology of neoliberalism" (Pritchard, 2020: 79).

Certainly, since the 1970s, governments of all party-political persuasion have rejected Keynesian ideals in favour of the adoption of liberal free market economies, a political model that some health researchers claim "make us sick" (Bambra & Schrecker, 2015). The extent to which political economies have shaped the cultures formed through, *and by*, the field of Arts in Health will be explored in this book over time and place. The usefulness of applying the label 'neoliberal' to this period of history is a topic to which, I hope, this account of the development of this field might speak. Those in Critical Public Health studies warn of the "peril of invoking neoliberalism" (Bell & Green, 2016), urging that this word not be used as a noun, so much as a verb to describe "partial and incomplete processes' (Ward & England, 2007). "Neoliberalism is neither omnipotent nor monolithic" a trade union organiser similarly affirms, claiming space for agency and action. "Instead of operating as a coherent ruling-class strategy, it is full of inconsistencies and contradictions" (Evans, 2022). Most recently, historians who query the periodisation of Britain's *Neoliberal Age since the 1970s* warn that when used as a "catch-all criticism", the term "simplifies links across different fields", "obscuring certain viewpoints" such as "a four nations perspective" (Davies et al., 2021: 2).

No less scrutiny has been given to other metanarratives used to characterise this period of history—those of multiculturalism and postcolonialism. Stuart Hall creation the field of Cultural Studies allowed for deeper articulations around how "Britain's black and brown populations visibly register a play of difference right across the face of British society" (Hall, 2001). It is now assuredly affirmed that "the composite nature of the British state" entails that "a simple presentation of a national history is not possible. Its national histories are several" (Bhambra, 2021: 5). I have tried to absorb related readings of culture and political economy into the writing this account of the niche, if also rather messy and sprawling, field of Arts in Health. I will attempt to show how certain policies have informed the formation of this field across time, especially those enacted across more than one nation, expressed by way of many different cultures and communities.

I use the descriptor 'Arts in Health' throughout this book with an awareness of the time-specific nature and use of this label.[14] It was adopted as a title around the millennium to replace the earlier idea of the 'healing arts' and the 'humanities in healthcare'. Different names reflect different "assumptions about the roots of ill-health and the way the arts can improve it" (White, 2009: 2). Taken together they are reflective of the "amorphous" and "shifting" status of this field (Broderick, 2011: 95). I respond to the need identified, by a researcher located within the field of Human Geography, not to fix meanings, but "talk afresh about arts-health as a combination of uncertain and contingent things to be explored" (Parr, 2017: 18).

This aim might be set alongside authors, researchers and practitioners within the field who detect "a recent resurgence of critical questions about arts and health" (Clift et al., 2021). One gave a "constructive critical" reading of the APPGAHW report, calling for "clearer" articulations of the field's "ideological commitments, underpinning beliefs about purpose and value" (Phillips, 2019: 21). These authors revive older critiques from previous decades around the poor quality of evidence (Belfiore, 2006) and the field's close relationship to governmental power (Mirza, 2006). Clift et al. stress the "need for robust critique" and question the extent to which current evidence shows that cultural engagement plays a "substantial role" in reducing "social and health inequalities" (ibid, p. 13).

While buoyed by the chance to join others in the task of any collective reappraisal, the terms of the critique deployed in this book are subtly different to those outlined above. I will be less concerned with either affirming or questioning "rigour" per se (Ravetz & Gregory, 2018), than to situate the political and economic contexts that have led to an unhealthy "obsession" with evidence-based research (Raw et al., 2012). Rather, this book will seek to examine how "interpretive practices" have become "part of the problem" (Banner, 2017: 16). I also draw on literatures within Critical Health Studies that examine health activism with the intention of "challenging the naturalization of progress narratives" (Diedrich, 2016: 13). Discourses developed within the Critical Medical Humanities point to the danger of "depoliticized" approaches to researching healthcare as these can serve, rather than undermine, harmful neoliberal models (Atkinson et al., 2016; Banner, 2021).

Taken together, critical discourses—arising out of many fields and disciplines—can be brought together to re-evaluate the field, throwing light on its "processes and pressures of connection, support, embedding, binding and generation" (Callard & Fitzgerald, 2015: 87). These reveal and show how "loose sets of institutions" have taken shape to become "visible and coherent sets of the interventions", with their own "journals, conferences, centres, funding streams and students" (ibid, p. 36). The terms on which shared understandings of the success and failure of the creative health agenda can thus be better assessed when seen as set of practices and institutions produced over time, through various "fields of contention" (Tilly, 2004; Tilly & Tarrow, 2015).

This book will re-visit histories surrounding the development of Arts in Health most particularly in response to the retrospective claim that it is field of practice best regarded as a social movement (Senior & Croall, 1993; White, 2009; Parkinson, 2011; Daykin, 2019). I respond to Lord Howarth's assertion that the NCCH "is not a model for the centre superimposed from on high," but one that has "emerged" out of "discussion among practitioners across the country". This book is aimed at a different audience to that targeted by the APPGAHW report: namely citizens, patients, creative practitioners and healthcare workers (those who bring about change in a different way to policymakers). I have tried to write it in a way that makes what has hitherto been a select, academic discussion, accessible for all.

Workers are the people most likely to comprise any collective social movement, those who might win improvements in working conditions or block unwelcome attacks on these. This distinction is important since "social movements can be engaged in either political or cultural conflicts meant to promote or oppose social change" (Della Porta & Diani, 2016: 21). Discussion amongst creative practitioners might include asking questions such as: how are we to judge what drives or delivers welcome social change across the arts and health sectors? How has the pandemic worked to enhance or detract from the creative health agenda through unjust structures or unequal allocation of resource? How have links been forged between different movements for social justice? What powers are currently being deployed, to win or block undesirable change?

Beyond the APPGAHW report's mission of advocacy, there appear to be few public platforms or forums to debate, qualify or raise such questions. There is a need to locate the points at which Arts in Health interventions risk becoming unhealthy (or uncreative) and to explore the values and ideologies that underpin assumptions.[15] The pandemic has prompted a radical questioning of political systems. This book aligns with those who believe that "never has it been more important to insist that another politics of life is possible" (Caduff, 2020). The pandemic has disturbed "temporalities and routines" making it uncertain when we might expect exceptional states to end and "normality" to resume (ibid, p. 475). Speculations around the 'health' of critique within the academy come from those who pinpoint the rise of authoritarian nationalism and new forms of censorship (Fassin, 2020), as well those who discern the end of the current Neoliberal age—or at least the "disruption and discrediting of the market ideal" (Davies & Gane, 2020: 3). An examination of how the moniker of 'creative health' had arrived at a celebratory moment of national consolidation in the UK—at a time of a tragic global crisis—appeared as a rich potential for writing a "history of the present" (Foucault, 1976). Through uncovering hidden conflicts, a re-evaluation of the phenomena of 'creative health' might be enabled (see note 14).

MYSTERIOUS ORIGINS

Though this book is not intended to provide a definitive account of the emergence of Arts in Health, it might act as a useful companion to those textbooks that do. A number of these have been published over the last five years (Clift & Camic, 2016; Stickley & Clift, 2017; Fancourt, 2017; Daykin, 2019a). These all suggest different beginning points and places at which Arts in Health practices can be seen to come together to form a discrete interdisciplinary field. In *Arts in Health: Designing and Researching Interventions* (Fancourt, 2017), Daisy Fancourt examines "the origins" of Arts in Health in prehistory relative to what she calls its "blossoming" in recent years (ibid, p. 2). Some of the limitation of taking an evidence-based research approach to the writing history is admitted by Fancourt in a defence she mounts towards an imagined critic. She guards the risk that her evidence can be seen as "circumspect" since she is limited by "lack of written evidence from the time" (ibid, p. 2). This is a problem solved when she moves on to later periods of history when texts, art works and documents become more readily available.

Her chapter on the history of Arts in Health extends into Paleolithic pre-history in order to demonstrate that no separation has *ever* existed between what are presented here as "interwoven" practices (Fancourt, 2017: 4). "The earliest sculptures ever made were created to support rituals around fertility and health...arts and health were very much interwoven from the beginning" (ibid, p. 5). Her assertion that the "birth of art was also the birth of arts in health" finds a mention in the APPGAHW report which describes the history provided by Fancourt as one that explores this topic "in some depth" (APPGAHW, 2017: 20). While covering a long period (40,000 years in 20 or so pages) it might be more accurate to describe this historical account as shallow. It moves swiftly from accounts of healing rituals in the ancient world, through to Medieval monasticism, before arriving at The Age of Enlightenment and the advent of the twentieth-century biomedicine.

The scholar who mounted one of the most rigorous and influential analyses of biomedical power, Michel Foucault, is cited just once by Fancourt in a paragraph on mental asylums. This reference is used to sound a rare bum note in what is otherwise presented as a harmonious narrative: "The arts were not always seen as positive for health", as they could lead to madness by way of "overindulgence of imagination exacerbated by the arts" (ibid, p. 7). At no other point in this narrative is this interwoven category unpicked. Rather, the guiding metaphor of "the bridge" is used on more than one occasion, albeit subject to potential cracks and tension: "the separation of medicine from the monastery did not mark the *breaking of the bridge*" (ibid, p. 8, *my italics*).

Such an interpretation of Arts in Health and its interdisciplinary nature are, I believe, deeply flawed. It assumes "prior wholeness as the condition of intersection" and goes against the need to "depart from the temporal frameworks and spatial strictures to which so many of today's practices of interdisciplinarity remain sadly tethered" (Fitzgerald & Callard, 2015: 38). Authors in the Medical Humanities point to missing "accounts of power" to explain how collaborations between those working out of different disciplines are produced through unequal (and unjust) structures of power, those brought about by unequal "financial, epistemic and cultural resources" (ibid, p. 97). What passes for 'interdisciplinarity' might merely offer ways to obscure and gloss over such points (ibid, p. 4).

Other authors writing on Arts in Health use the 'inter' descriptor by way of more recent accounts of the field's formation. In *The Oxford Textbook of Creative Arts, Health and Well-being: international perspectives on practice policy and research*, the editors recognise that the "idea that the creative arts have a direct role in the area of people suffering from illness" has a "long history" one that "appears in cultures throughout the world" (Clift & Camic, 2016, p. 7). But only since the beginning of the twentieth century has "serious attention" been given the "potential of the arts in therapeutic and healthcare interventions". As for the reason why serious attention was only given at this time, the authors merely speculate that it will be for "future historians to reflect on the factors and influences accounting for the growth of interest" (Clift & Camic, 2016: 7). They further quote Lord Howarth's diagnosis of a "Pathology of the West" through which Arts in Health practitioners are cast in the role of "heretics and radicals", those who "challenge dominant values and conventional policies" (ibid, p. 8).

In *Arts, Health and Wellbeing: A Theoretical Inquiry for Practice* (Stickley & Clift, 2017) the same editor (working with a different colleague) locates the field's "emergence" in more recent decades. In the preface they write: "This inter-disciplinary field has emerged...over the last 20–30 years" (Stickley & Clift, 2017: 1). A single sentence acknowledges the oddness of this growth taking place in a decade marked by austerity and a period of deep cuts to public spending in the UK. The editors appear to strike a note of surprise, as much as satisfaction, when they note how "despite the challenges of economic cut-backs, the field of practice has thrived". They offer a brief speculation as to why this might be the case: "perhaps largely because of a groundswell of grassroots artists that believe in the importance of the work" (ibid, p. 1).

The idea that Arts in Health is a social movement informed by a "groundswell" of support is most directly addressed in Norma Daykin's recent textbook, *Arts, Health and Well-Being: A Critical Perspective on Research, Policy and Practice* (Daykin, 2019). Here, there is a full and frank acknowledgement of "non neutrality and the role of political governance regulation and social action" in the creation of the field (Daykin, 2019: 1). Daykin also acknowledges the limitation of evidence-based approaches, arguing that new theories are now needed to address "strategic questions", listed here as "the relationship between evidence, policy and practice, as well as practical issues of propagation and scale in arts, health and wellbeing" (Daykin, 2019: 4) . Social movement theory is presented as "useful" for further research in that it can "help to unpack challenging questions about the nature of evidence by highlighting their political and moral basis" (ibid, p. 45). Daykin charts those who have used this descriptive term over time (Del Castillo et al., 2017; Parkinson, 2015;

RSPH, 2013) and writes a key passage on why different actors have chosen to present the field as such, listing very different motivations.

> Some are motivated by personal experience, while others seek to resolve specific professional or clinical problems, and others are focused on strategic policy issues and resources. A few operate from commercial interests, while many emphasise a rights-based approach to arts, culture and wellbeing, advocating socially engaged arts practice as a way of challenging elitist notions of 'high art' in favour of community involvement and social inclusion (ibid, p. 48).

Daykin is shy in explicitly stating her own commitment, merely concluding that Arts in Health can indeed be usefully seen as a social movement. Yet she too still speaks of "overcoming divisions" by way of "bridges" (ibid, p. 2) with little further acknowledgement that knowledge exchange comes about through conflictual processes. This is the case even while she refers to how social movements have been interpreted by way of contentious politics—what Charles Tilly describes as the "continuous interaction between challengers and power holders" who together comprise "third parties such as repressive forces, allies, competitors," as well as "citizenry as a whole" (Tilly, 1999: 270). Daykin plays down the usefulness of his Tilly's theory in relation to the field, observing that "recent thinking" has "shifted away" towards a more "nuanced" understanding of the energies generated by social movements, framed less by "combative" positions (Daykin, 2019: 48). I propose that Tilly's framing remains all too relevant amid rising fears for the health of Western democracies in the face of populist social movements. As a reviewer of Tilly's most recent work observes, "contentious politics" can aid "the quest for a non-violent world, where dissent can be aired and a form of agonistic democracy nourished" (Long, 2016: 1).

These, then, are some of the speculative origination stories told about the field of Arts in Health and its recent blossoming and growth. They are told by way of authors published by Oxford and Cambridge imprints that themselves lend these narratives a certain scholastic authority.

WALES AND NORTHERN ENGLAND

The questions raised above are ones I had been thinking about before the pandemic, through a three-year long period of research towards a PhD (Williams, 2019). This was undertaken at Manchester Metropolitan University between 2016 and 2019 (though I lived in North Wales throughout this time). Much of the material for this book has been taken from my literature review which included an overview of critical undercurrents within Arts in Health over a 20-year period. This provided a preamble to an anthropological study of contemporary understandings of creative health, how 'creativity', 'health' and 'place' were being understood and interpreted at a local authority level across North Wales and the North of England. Greater Manchester's city leaders had struck a secret 'devo-deal' with HM Treasury in 2015, the first-time local authorities had gained control over healthcare budgets since the NHS was established in 1948. In this way, my research encompassed a parallel understanding of Arts in Health, how it was understood in the past, as well as in the present.

Through this, I came to recognise how *tone-deaf* celebratory notes (such those detailed above) were not odd blips but had been frequently sounded by actors working in the field. In the years when policies of austerity were introduced in the UK, for example, one of the first people to write an account of the development of Arts in Health wondered "if the future is really so bright we need to wear sunglasses?" (White, 2014). The insistence on bright futures in the face of dark backdrops promoted me to look more deeply into what White went on to name as the field's unethical direction or "misdirection" (ibid, p. 2).

Before undertaking this body of research for a PhD, I was involved in developing and running Arts in Health projects. I grew up in South Wales before coming to London, firstly to train as an artist, later moving into gallery education. My motivation to raise questions from within the field is one that principally arises out of care and attention for the work and those whom it touches. I have promoted the creative health 'agenda' myself. One of the projects I instigated, *Creative Families* (SLG, 2015), saw local authority agencies refer parents with mental health needs to work with artists. Evaluation findings from this project are included in the APPGAHW report. I further co-hosted a public talk in 2018 in partnership with Cardiff University to profile the APPGAHW report in Wales (see note 15). My aim with this book, then, is to open up discussion amongst wider publics rather than close them down through authoritative last words. Critique, not as "the practice of destruction and naysaying" but as a "revolution at the level of procedure without which we cannot secure rights of dissent and processes of legitimation" (Butler, 2009; 773).

The following chapters will explore some of the histories of contention surrounding the development of diverse Arts in Health formations across various social movements, forms of art practice and academic disciplines alike. It is written from a partial position, askance one might say, from a Welsh perspective. The book's title is a deliberate provocation on the idea that creative health is an idea whose "time has come". It alludes to Gwyn Alf Williams' study of Welsh history titled *When Was Wales?* (1979). Williams wrote playfully on the how the Welsh were "difficult to identify" since all nations were "made not born" (ibid, p. 6).

Others have since riffed on Williams work by way of odd temporalities to ask *Why Wales Never Was* (Brooks, 2017) or claimed Wales as England's "first and final colony" (Price, 2016). In recent years, perspectives on cultural plurality within Wales have emerged (Chetty, 2022) alongside accounts of neoliberalism as a distinctive "Welsh way" of life (Evans et al., 2021). These simultaneously highlight the shortcomings of devolution and dangers of ethno-nationalism, pointing towards diverse, sustainable futures for Welsh culture by way of a re-imagined (often independent) Welsh nation. A more careful "forensic focus" is now drawn between different forms of 'colonialism' (internal and external) since it is more fully and rightly acknowledged that the Welsh were "not the victims of colonial oppression but active participants in the imperial project" (Owens, 2022).

While there might be a consensus on the point that the origins of Arts in Health cannot be conclusively located in any single nation, one fact also in need of acknowledgement is that claims around the 'birth' of Arts in Health in Prehistoric society find expression in contemporary political contexts in the UK. "Think of the caveman!" was how the Chief Executive of Arts Council Wales (Nick Capaldi) urged the Minister of Health for Wales (Vaughan Gethin) to justify and celebrate his support for a *Concordat for Arts in Health* launched in 2017.[16] Such references, perhaps lifted all too lightly from Arts in Health textbooks, lend legitimacy to such interpretations through their repetition in UK policy circles. It is an adoption of prehistory, we can note, that has been queried by some anthropologists who throw doubt on whether any explanatory rationale for advanced capitalist societies can be gleaned from "cranial remains and the occasional piece of knapped flint" (Graeber & Wengrow, 2021: 81).

Capaldi further quoted the words of a fictional academic—Professor Dumbledore, of Harry Potter fame—in a clumsy attempt to popularise the case for Arts in Health. "Ah, music, a magic beyond all we do hear!"[17] Cave paintings, we can note, also appear in presentations given by the United Nations (UN) representative for Arts in Health—a supra-national body which commissioned Daisy Fancourt to provide an extensive evidence review in 2019 (Fancourt & Finn, 2019). At different levels of governance then—both supra, national and devolved—it is possible to see the uses to which Arts in Health histories draw on reassuring, repeated emblems, applicable across all time, all place, all people.

As part of this genealogical inquiry, I refer to a (non-fictional) Professor of Gender Studies, Lisa Diedrich, who has made a useful study of health activism which examines the nature of "pre-histories" and "pre-conditions" whereby certain "substances" come into being (Diedrich, 2016: 12). In her book, *Indirect Action, Schitzophrenia, Epilespy, Aids and the Course of Health Activism*, Foucault's idea of 'histories of the present' is raised alongside feminist interpretations of history to show how "echoes" perform "not exact" repetitions of the past that can aid "serious analytical work" (Scott, 1991: 286). Diedrich then goes on to listen for 'echoes' in how health activisms were enacted in New York City in the 1980s. This was a time when this city became the site for many forms of political resistance, both direct and indirect, to the AIDS epidemic and its deadly impacts.

I have also taken inspiration from Camille Robcis' book *Disalienation* (Robcis, 2021) which charts the rise and fall of 'institutional psychotherapy' through its emergence after the Second World War to its abandonment in the 1970s. Though she begins her study at the site of its first expression—the Saint Elan Hospital in France—she does not to claim any single place as "sole origin". Rather, she explores "the role that a particular setting, or context can have in fostering ideas" (Robcis, 2021: 13). Robcis gives a thrilling account of how French theory was informed by displaced doctors fleeing German occupation and Nazi ideology from other European countries.

In conclusion, then, I do not seek to situate Arts in Health here as a 'British' phenomenon. Rather, I aim to plot the some-place and some-time over the everywhere and has-been-forever. Multi-national (and regional) perspectives allow histories of division to be explored, those fostered by economic inequality as well as those that reflect cultural difference. They allow a history of Arts in Health to be considered by way of the

UK's exit from the European Union as well as the UK's longer Imperial past. Shifting borders reflect the UK's mutually related role as a 'Union' and an 'Empire'. When taken alone "as the unit of analysis" and "not the wider empire, or imperial state", a misleading idea of the UK as a self-supporting unit is mistakenly perpetuated (Bhambra, 2021: 13). "Relations of extraction", Gurminda Bhambra argues, can all too easily be confused and conflated with the welfare state's "relations of redistribution" (ibid, 5). "The territorial boundaries of the British state, as well as organizational structure, have never been congruent with what many see as the imagined nation" (ibid, p. 5). Thus the expanding and contracting terms that constitute UK citizenship seem central to any discussion of inequality in relation to the formation of the field of Arts in Health.

The first ever National Network for Arts in Health (NNAH) was formed at a time when acts of devolution were passed (between 1997 and 2000). I propose that this may be not so coincidental a fact as might, as first, be assumed. Perceptions of the unequal treatment of communities living in the home nations acted as a powerful driver for the referendums which allowed devolved government to come into being. Despite the early hope invested in devolution, a growing number of people in Wales, Scotland and Northern Ireland now see how devolved power might just as easily be withdrawn, as it was granted, at the discretion of those sitting in post-Brexit Westminster.

Greater awareness of the skewed, unequal and shifting distributions of British state can also help us query common accounts of the international flavour of Arts in Health—those written by UK authors whose focus tends to be on inequality in a global context. "The so-called lifestyle diseases of the first world are now increasingly afflicting the developing world", Helen Chatterjee and Guy Noble state in their introduction to *Museums, Health and Well-being* (Chatterjee & Noble, 2017: ix). "Globalization means the exportation of poor health from rich countries to less well-off nations". Such emphases tend to position the UK as a rich, coherent nation, rather than a set of divided territories 'united' through histories of extractive capitalism. Broad iterations of "*our* heritage", as used in this book, serve to obscure the fact that some cultural heritages emerge through erasure, and so must be seen as healthy (for some) but altogether less healthy (for others).

Today, poorer areas of the UK are frequently characterised as those 'left behind' by both the state and the market. But they were cast and understood in the 1970s as peripheral "fringes" brought about by "internal colonialism" (Hechter, 1975). Assumptions of the efficacy of capitalist systems to redress inequality risk endorsing a "view that efficient markets will level all ethnic and racial differences and bring about cultural unity" (ibid, p. xiii). They leave unaddressed exploitative histories, not least those pertaining to the NHS as the benefactor of "colonial legacies of value extraction" (Bhattacharyya et al., 2020: 73). These legacies have been entrenched in Wales, and the UK more widely, with "an economic model and social settlement built on hundreds of years of fossil fuel and Global South exploitation" (Jones, 2022).

Health 'gaps' in rates of mortality (Marmot, 2017) have been exacerbated by the pandemic as previous protocols—particularly those that respect political and cultural difference—have been abandoned, it will be argued. In the wake of exit of the UK from the EU, there has been a reaffirmation of 'muscular' unionism whereby the political autonomy granted to the home nations has been once again thrown into question: devolution was 'Tony Blair's biggest mistake' (Johnson, 2020). This has gone hand in hand with racist rhetoric that casts all "foreign bodies" as potential threat to the integrity of Great Britain (Napier, 1996, 2020).

External 'threats' have been conjured and aligned with internal ones since the onset of the COVID-19 pandemic. Alongside President Trump's labelling of virus as "The China virus", one English media pundit dubbed calls for political independence, made by Scottish and Welsh political groupings, "the Celtic virus" (Jenkins, 2021). This is surely as cruel a metaphor, as it is inaccurate, given that parts of post-industrial Wales had the highest mortality rates per capita of anywhere else in the UK at the height of the pandemic—a vulnerability made possible by conditions of poverty stretching back many decades. Such 'metaphors of illness' (Sontag, 1978) are not beyond the scope of what constitutes our understanding of Arts in Health. Rather they show up the field's dense historical entanglement with the construction of Britishness and the spatial inequalities that constitute the basis of the UK, both past and present.

ORGANISATION OF CHAPTERS

Chapters proceed more of less chronologically to explore recurring themes and arguments relating to what Arts in Health (and latterly creative health) might constitute. I have titled chapters not by decades but by the names given to creative (health) practitioners across these different periods of time. As well as tracing histories across post-war decades, attention to

contemporary interpretations of these histories are simultaneously provided to throw into relief the uses to which these narratives are being put
today. Certain contentions repeat. I leave some of the work (and hopefully
the pleasure too) of detecting echoes and their distortion to the reader,
while others I spell out more explicitly.

Each chapter is loosely organised around debates between individuals
who either practiced, theorised or engaged in the production of Arts in
Health. I lean heavily towards the visual arts, whilst also giving a focus to
'social art practice' as these reflect my own area of knowledge. The following two chapters take a wide focus, before narrowing into a more granular
study of how Arts in Health was instituted over the last 20 years, in
Chap. 4.

Following on from this introduction, Chap. 2 examines the (pre) and
post-war period to examine the national basis on which the foundational
institution of the NHS was created, contrasting this with the promise
offered by regional devolution more recently. Chapter 3 focuses on how
the creation of Arts in Health was informed by international social movements in the 1960s and 70s. These challenged the over-extension of biomedical authority as exercised by way of the state as well as the market. I
discuss of the ways in which social hierarchies were deconstructed through
the emergence of 'counter' and 'sub' cultures. The work of community
artists was funded by the local state, which in the 1980s offered scope for
their demands to be met through democratic processes exercised at this
level of government.

Chapter 4 charts the most recent set of networks and alliances that
constitute the formation of Arts in Health by way of a various texts—
including a declaration, charter, prospectus and manifesto—before returning to the APPGAHW report and its extensive evidence-base. Two
influential models are profiled, those cited as exemplifying an Arts in
Health approach; the Bromley-by-Bow Health Centre in London and
START in Manchester. These two organisations reveal how nuanced strategies, involving market integration, were adopted to offer alternate and
supplementary provision to that of the welfare state.

A final chapter examines where critique has been imagined to reside
within Arts in Health practices and how and when these might have
become subsumed or rendered redundant. Attention is given to the most
recent spatialisation of the field as a possible 'accelerator' in attempts to
'level-up' the North of England. This suggests that the unfulfilled hope of
Arts in Health rests on a longer failure to adequately address or reverse

widening geographies of inequality: one linked to the spread of neoliberal models of governance adopted at all tiers and levels, the common adoption of a type of "politics that makes us sick" (Bambra & Schrecker, 2015).

A final brief note on images: I use these to illustrate salient issues in each chapter; the statue of slave trader Edward Colston toppled by the city's residents, in Chap. 1; designs for good living and images of collective endeavour in Chap. 2. The human body made subject to structural violence and 'cuts', in Chap. 3; illustrations of rebellion and recovery in Chap. 4. Just as I begin this book with an image of a fallen statue, so I end with those retained and re-erected, in Manchester in Chap. 5: (that of the anti-abolitionist Prime Minister, William Gladstone, alongside Communist Party founder, Friedrich Engels.)

Ultimately, the aim of this book is not to condemn or endorse the revised concept of creative health, to write neither a dismissive critique nor a hagiography. Rather, it is to provide the means to better locate points of failure and success for the future, by way of how they have been understood in the past. I hope any reader might find their own place amongst the different political, social and artistic commitments set out across the times and places navigated here. As Nick Crossley argues, social movements always involve a "variety of forms of know-how, dispositions and schemas" (Crossley, 2005: 22). These lead to "taken-for-granted knowledges of the history, heroes, demons and martyrs of their causes" (ibid, p. 23). It is towards a reappraisal of assumptions and this field's key figures and guiding metaphors that we can now directly turn.

NOTES

1. This lockdown extended across all four nations (England, Scotland, Northern Ireland and Wales). After March 2020, lockdowns would differ in duration across these jurisdictions and tiers of devolved government. They would also be imposed at different times within different regions of England too.
2. APPGAHW Chair Lord Howarth and the Acting Director of the NCCH, Alex Coulter, are quoted in an article in Arts Professional. https://www.artsprofessional.co.uk/news/national-centre-creative-health-mainstream-arts-health-and-social-care.
3. The report was researched and drafted by Dr Rebecca Gordon-Nesbitt, Research Fellow at Kings College London. The report's overall content was edited by those comprising the APPG Inquiry committee of which Lord Howarth was Chair.

4. May assumed office from David Cameron following the Brexit referendum result, which resulted in his resignation.
5. Michael Marmot was invited to endorse the report which acknowledges that it "extended" his work. The previous omission of the arts as representative of a positive social determinant of health is characterised in the report as a "blind spot" (APPGAHW, 2017: 50).
6. The report quotes a contributor to one of the APPG roundtables, Professor Richard Parish, on this point (APPGAHW, 2017: 30).
7. They recounted the cautionary tale of austerity-hit Greece and posed the question: How many 'UK arts organisations can honestly say that their local communities would erect the barricades to defend them?'
8. For more information on STPs, see https://www.independent.co.uk/voices/biggest-change-nhs-you-ve-never-heard-a7218536.html.
9. In a launch event which can be accessed on the website: https://www.youtube.com/watch?v=o6DEHuDVCIA.
10. Trump refers here to the killing of an anti-racist protestor at Charlottesville. https://www.washingtonpost.com/politics/2020/05/08/very-fine-people-charlottesville-who-were-they-2/
11. Such as in Winnipeg, Canada, where both a statue of Queen Victoria and Queen Elizabeth II were defaced and toppled. See The Art Newspaper. https://www.theartnewspaper.com/2021/07/02/crowds-topple-statues-of-queen-victoria-and-elizabeth-ii-in-winnipeg-amid-anger-over-deaths-of-indigenous-children.
12. The vaccine administration was differently managed by the respective NHS services across England, Wales Scotland and Northern Ireland. But all benefitted from being public bodies delivering a universal healthcare service.
    See the government report, *Coronavirus: Lessons Learned to Date* (2021). https://www.gov.uk/government/publications/coronavirus-lessons-learned-to-date-report-government-response
13. https://www.gov.uk/government/news/new-legal-protection-for-england-s-heritage.
14. Foucault describes his study of medical knowledge, *The Birth of the Clinic*, as an 'archaeology'. The phrase 'history of the present' is used in his book, *Discipline and Punish* (1977), but also appears in his earlier book, *The Order of Things* (1970). See David Garland's paper of 2015, titled: What is a "history of the present"? On Foucault's genealogies, Punishment & Society 2014, Vol. 16(4) 365–384.
15. See this blog https://www.artshealthcrn.com/post/an-essential-vaccine-cardiff-uk-ahecrn-event.

16. Devolution does not receive any mention in this book, nor does 'place' as such though Salford is mentioned as one area where social movement approaches have been adopted, one of six 'vanguard sites' supported to do so by the NHS programme, Health as a Social Movement.
17. For more details of this event, see my PhD thesis (Williams, 2019: 168).

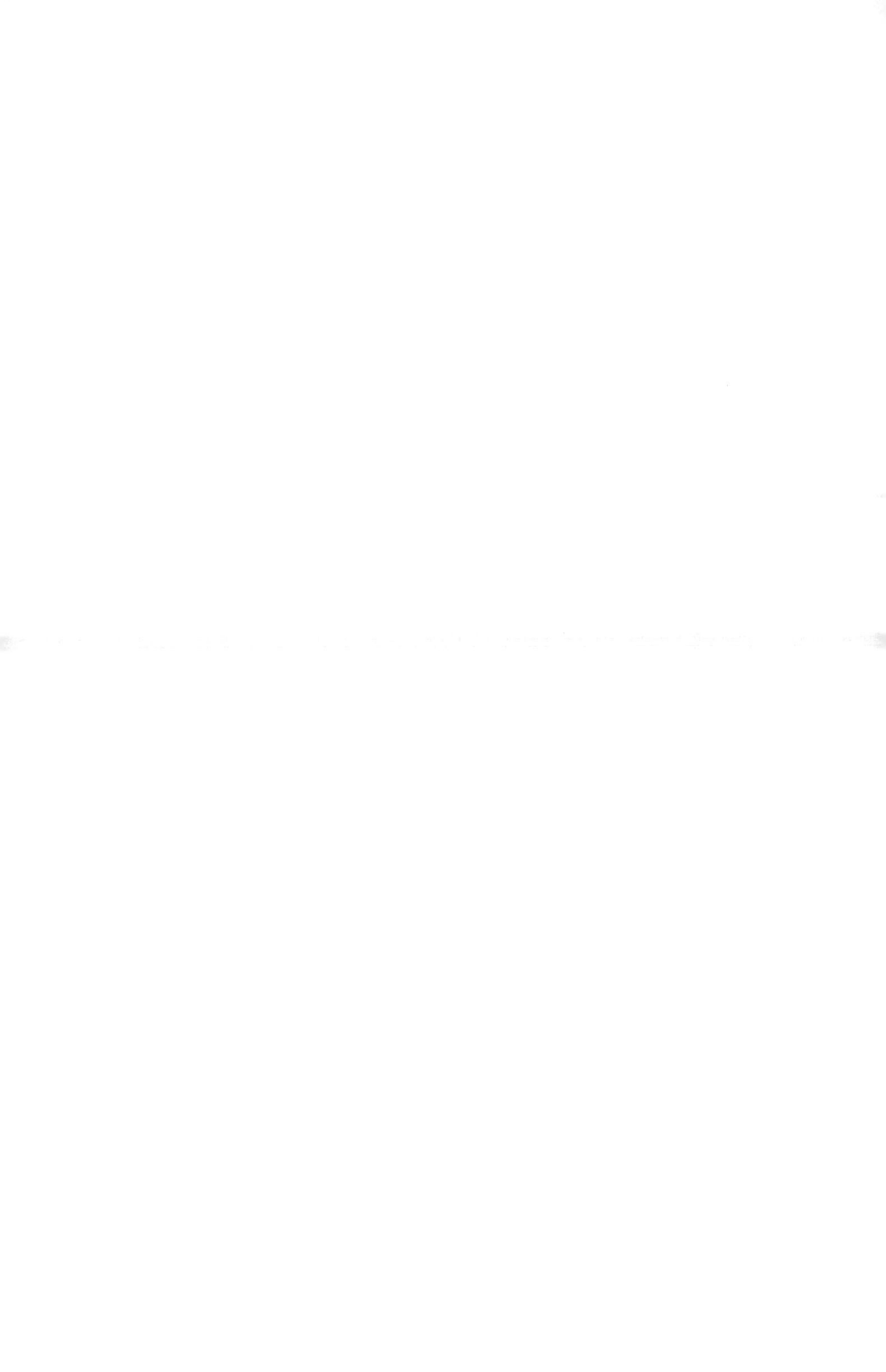

CHAPTER 2

Dreamers, Sufferers, Builders

The British nation state and the development of the field of Arts in Health are linked through the institutional formation of what was, and is still called today, the *National Health Service* (NHS). In this chapter, the pre- and post-war decades will be examined as a "fomenting" period for the emergence of this category of art practice (Diedrich, 2016: 10). Despite being made subject to successive waves of reform, the NHS is an institution whose foundational values and early symbolisms continue to "haunt" the present (Fisher, 2009).[1] Forged through sharply opposing political ideologies, some of the ongoing contentions that any discussion of the NHS sets in play in relation to Arts in Health include the funding of preventative health relative to healthcare services designed to treat illness; the role of the state in setting the terms of British citizenship; as well as the role of personal and collective agency in the pursuit of health beyond medical provision alone.

WHAT'S IN A NAME?

The first contention centres on the question of 'health' and how we define it. WHO affirmed a definition in the same year that the NHS was established in 1948: "A state of complete physical, mental and social wellbeing and not merely the absence of disease or infirmity" (WHO, 1948). Through questioned by some doctors working today as an "outdated", even "utopian" ideal (Misselbrook, 2014), this remains the definition most favoured in Arts in Health literatures (and the APPGAHW report) as it "embraces a positive and holistic understanding of what it means to be healthy in body, mind and community" (APPGAHW, 2017: 16). This expansive definition is preferred over any which use biomedical criteria alone or those that that make too sharp a distinction between states of 'sickness' and 'health'.[2] Neither static, nor binary, these are states that naturally fluctuate over the lifespan (Aronovsky, 1979).

By way of such distinction, the NHS acronym has frequently been cast as a misnomer. "For all practical purposes, it is a National Sickness Service that treats people once they are ill" (Greer, 2004). This is an interpretation of the role of the NHS increasingly supported by a host of UK civic organisations, such as *The Health Creation Alliance*, whose voices find a place within the APPGAHW report. The rising financial cost of healthcare, relative to ill-health, is foregrounded in many of these commentaries. One public health official pointed to unsustainable levels of investment between resources allocated to support public health as opposed to those allocated for the treatment of illness in 2015. 'Forget Privatization' the (former) Chief Medical Officer of Scotland urged, it's more important to enable the creation of a "well-being service" than resource an ever expanding "sickness service," (Burns, 2015: 1).[3] Though emphasising the obvious benefit of prevention over cure, such re-namings have also been criticised as "facile sloganeering", an interpretation of causality that "systematically ignores the implications of the rhetoric" in specific political and economic contexts (Heath, 2007: 334). "A reconstituted National Health Service that prioritises prevention of sickness would fail all those who are ill now" (ibid, p. 335).

Leaving aside the 'H', further contentions centre on the 'N in the NHS' (Bivens & Crane, 2017). Most obviously, the "NHS has been divided into politically autonomous health systems since 1998" due to acts of devolution (Greer, 2016). Detailing developments prior to this point, Scott Greer asserts that "in effect", there was only a brief period that that "all national health service systems were directly owned and run by central government" (ibid, p. 20). He points out that "Scotland's NHS was born at the same time as the English NHS in 1948", while "The Welsh NHS was only carved out of the English NHS in 1969", part of what he calls a "NHS family of systems" that developed prior to formal acts of devolution in the late 1990s (ibid, p. 18). The APPGAHW report does not dwell on these finer points, taking a brisk approach to differences across political systems established over time and place. Whilst acknowledging "proprieties", a wish to breach political boundaries is declared:

> In deference to the proprieties of devolution, the recommendations we make as an all-party group at Westminster are addressed to people making decisions in England, but we hope they may have useful applicability in the other nations of the UK. (APPGAHW, 2017: 6)

These "other nations" are commonly taken to comprise the 'National' character of the NHS, one that is popularly (if inaccurately) presented as a uniting institution that subsumes internal division. Former war victories have been invoked to project a sense of unity. The Secretary of State for Health spoke of the NHS taking on a "heroic fight" against COVID-19 in July 2020, for example, using battle metaphors. He compared his own leadership style (and that of NHS managers) to Admiral Nelson at the Battle of Trafalgar when "the navy was heavily outnumbered" with ships' captains "hamstring by the fog of war" (Hancock, 2020). Similarly, the "blitz spirit" of the Second World War (taken as a psychological state of resilience) was further evoked by Hancock, since everyone "pulled together in one gigantic national effort". The NHS was repeatedly cast as defender of the British nation.[4]

The post-war years, however, were not marked by the victory over Nazi Germany in Europe alone. They also marked the loss of imperial territories once held under British colonial rule. National independence movements successfully won their freedom from Britain in these decades: India and Pakistan in 1947; Ghana in 1957; Nigeria and Somalia in 1960; Sierra Leone in 1961; Uganda in 1963 and Kenya in 1964. These relinquishments mark a significant, if often overlooked, aspect of how the NHS was created, not least through the recruitment of health workers from the newly created Commonwealth territories. People in the West Indies were encouraged to work as NHS staff, a new healthcare body created in the same year as the first *Windrush* ship arrived in the UK from these islands.

Post-colonial histories of the NHS, one historian asserts, point to "the limits of belonging in a multi-ethnic welfare state" (Bivens, 2015). Efforts to assimilate migrant workers, Roberta Bivens insightfully notes, were predicated on a "normative agenda of incorporation into a fluid, but supposedly singular 'national culture'" (ibid, p. 9). Historian David Olusoga likewise argues that the NHS was "a system that needed them *(migrant workers)* but didn't always want them". He examined "hidden histories" of racism in the NHS for a BBC programme on this topic aired in 2021, one which saw him interview Irish nurses alongside those from the Caribbean.[5] Olusoga used the possessive title, *"Our* International NHS" (my italics) with intent to speak of a more complex set of inclusions/exclusions than any single 'national' narrative alone can establish.

Yet despite these necessary qualifications, the NHS acronym retains common usage by general publics and politicians of all party-political persuasion. Cultural theorists have suggested that this is reflective of an affective attachment to projected values. The NHS is "imbued" with "egalitarian" principles (Bivens & Crane, 2017: 12). The welfare state is seen as reflective of the British character, one which holds up "ideals of fair play" as the Liberal economist William Beveridge originally expressed this sentiment in his 1942 report (Beveridge, 1942: 172). Less attention has been given, until recently, to the eugenicist beliefs which informed Beveridge's use of the term 'The British race' in the same report (Shilliam, 2018). Such selective attentions reveal how the Welfare state was informed by Modernity and egalitarian desires, whilst also continuing to be reflective of "deeply embedded attitudes and traditions – about race, 'civilization' and health" (Bivens, 2015: 12).

The role of the NHS as a virtuous symbol in the national psyche has been expressed through diverse art forms and graphic representation over time, those which have informed perceptions of how "multicultural" British society is, was, or could be (Hall, 2001). "Visual sources… clearly indicate that the possessive community implied by the repeated phrases 'your NHS' and 'our NHS' was assumed and intended to be a homogenous 'British public' that even in 1948 certainly did not exist" (Bivens, 2015). It further acted as a potent trope, for example, when performed to a global audience at the opening ceremony of the Olympic Games in London in 2012. As part of this event, the NHS logo was lit up in fireworks, part of a spectacular mass performance which saw volunteer doctors and nurses joyfully dance around beds in a choreographed display of care. (This followed an earlier sequence showing clips from The Four Nations Rugby tournament, projected against the sound of choirs singing anthems of each of the four nations.)

Some journalists watching Danny Boyle's extravagant production interpreted it as 'a love letter to Britain', while others cautioned against the use of NHS iconography in this celebratory context (including the Minister for Health at the time, it was later revealed).[6] "The idea of the Health Service as a beacon for the world is, bluntly, a national self-delusion", a columnist in

The Times objected (Gilligan, 2012). His point finds support amongst those who look back today on Boyle's portrayal of historic social movements to critique them as safely anodyne. Boyle encouraged the British public "to remember the Chartists but not the Mau Mau; the suffragettes not the British Black Panther Party" (Bhattacharyya et al., 2020: 73). These movements were not included in this iteration of "progressive patriotism" it is noted by authors keen to challenge the revival of this notion today (by a Labour Party led by Kier Starmer). "A future Labour government should embrace patriotism" (Nandy, 2021).

Boyle's cultural interpretation of the NHS as a British institution found fulsome welcome, it can be noted, by one prominent Arts in Health advocate writing at the time. Blogging in his capacity as the Director of Research at Durham University's *Centre of Medical Humanities*, Mike White appropriated this part of the Olympic ceremony as a "massive declaration for arts and health", claiming it showed how they made "perfect bedfellows" in this instance (White, 2013: 1). Culture was shown to be the "bedrock of healthcare... expressed with a sweeping confidence that the viewing public would understand" (ibid, p. 1). White's comments present an interesting perspective on the role of popular culture in promoting the idea of Arts in Health since they point to a gap between 'expert' understandings and general publics in need of easy explanation about the benefit of this relation.

In his book, *Arts Development in Community Health: a Social Tonic*, (2009), White is one of the few chroniclers of the recent history of the field of Arts in Health to credit the post-war period as one which saw the awakening of a new type of consciousness:

> ...an awareness of the need to mobilise public participation in preventative health strategies that are socialising goes back to the very foundation of Britain's National Health Service. (White, 2009: 3)

He identifies this moment as one that reveals links between 'socialising' art forms and those able to foster community health. Arts development can act as an effervescent "social tonic", he affirms in this book. His hope, on seeing the Olympic celebration, was that it could help "breach the sceptical barrier of healthcare policy and admit arts in health as *a small-scale global phenomenon*" (ibid, my italics). This presents a curiously modest, yet expansive characterisation of Arts in Health, one to which we will return (in Chap. 5).

Such warmly unifying affirmations could be seen as building on the observation that the NHS is "the closest thing the English have to a religion".[7] This phrase is often repeated by those who claim the NHS as an unhealthy emotional attachment, one that sets it beyond any critical assessment, let alone moral reproach. Any sense of prohibition that surrounds criticism of the NHS has been flipped in recent years by those keen to break what has been cast as a sacrilegious taboo. "We love the NHS so much it is killing us" a health policy officer for a right-of-centre think tank asserted in a 2016 (Griffiths, 2016).[8] Nuanced debate on the merits and drawbacks of the NHS is essential—one local actor working to promote Arts in Health in Manchester believes—since polarisations can quickly descend into unconstructive "battle grounds".[9]

Socialist Values

The contentious public discourses outlined above go some way to explaining the reticence shown in the APPGAHW report towards commenting on what the problem of "healthcare culture" in the NHS was, is, or might involve opposing (or be seen to oppose). But there are other reasons to be found for this restrained critique in a closer study of the original political movements that informed the creation of the NHS. For it was in the (pre)war years, in the late 1930s and early 1940s, that "the story of the NHS became the story of the Labour Party" (Broxton, 2017).

Architect of the NHS, Aneurin Bevan, brought socialist values to his task, beliefs deeply informed by his upbringing in South Wales. Radical politics flourished in the mining communities living here at this time. Social lives centred around chapels, choirs, libraries and working men's institutes—institutions that enabled political education. "Welsh nonconformist traditions and social practices had instilled in mining communities a desire for and belief in reading, culture and self-education" (Baggs, 2003: 116). A sense of social and intellectual independence led to these places being portrayed as potential sources of communist revolution in the 1920s and 1930s. One national tabloid newspaper, for example, dubbed the mining village of Maerdy in the Rhondda, 'Little Moscow'—a slander which townsfolk reappropriated as a badge of pride.[10]

This upbringing equipped Bevan with an intuitive understanding of how different facets of community life might combine though fiscal and social policy. After the war, Health was a policy priority which was nested amongst a wider programme of social reforms imagined across all government departments—including education, culture and housing (the latter's remit being one Bevan also oversaw as part of his cabinet brief). It was in his capacity as Minister for Housing that Bevan declared his mission to re-build post-war Britain by way of social egalitarianism. "We have been the dreamers, we have been the sufferers, and now, we are the builders" he asserted in an 1945 election speech. (Bevan, 1946).

His vision for the NHS was situated within the overarching premise of the welfare state outlined in the Beveridge report of 1942. But it was Bevan who demanded a healthcare system equally accessible and free to all regardless of where people lived. "We shall promise every citizen in this country the same standard of service" (Bevan, 1946). Bevan saw a risk, one that some contemporary researchers also foreground, that "health localism exacerbates the very divide which it should heal" (Harrop & Phibbs, 2017: 4).

His vision would be fulfilled on the back of a landslide Labour Party victory in 1945. But it also rested on a more intimate victory over his cabinet colleague, Herbert Morrison. Morrison had argued that any new health service should be run through local authorities, a move Bevan opposed:

> Bevan understood that the local authority model could not provide what he saw as fundamental to socialised medicine, equal access and treatment irrespective of where one lived and irrespective of arbitrary historical boundaries. (Stewart, 2017: 8)

Dr Stephen Taylor, influential in developing Labour Party health policy in the late 1930s, raised the point that the "municipal needs of the poor areas are greater than those of the rich, so that rates (i.e. local taxation) fall heaviest on those least able to bear them" (Taylor, 1979). London boasted good healthcare services, he claimed, because it held within its boundary many affluent areas able to subsidise poorer ones. His assertion was supported by Morrison who proposed the London Council health model on this basis. But Bevan rejected this model for the same reason Morrison championed it: poorer areas could also boast relatively good health outcomes when resource was distributed fairly and all residents were taxed in (equal) proportion to their income.

It was Bevan's national vision that won the day based on his experience of a template of mutual aid first adopted in his hometown of Tredegar.

Miners had long operated a *Medical Aid Society* here, one that employed doctors, a surgeon, pharmacist, physiotherapist, dentist and district nurse. Members paid extra to benefit from hospital treatment and, by the mid-1940s, the society provided healthcare for 22,800 of the town's 24,000 inhabitants. In the concise words of Tudor Hart (activist doctor of the 1970s), the Tredegar model allowed miners to "tax themselves" and create "their own income tax".[11] Bevan became chair of the *Medical Aid Society* at a young age and so was intimate with this system's many benefits, one he wanted "to export to the world" (Broxton, 2017). "All I am doing is extending to the entire population of Britain the benefits we had in Tredegar for a generation or more" (ibid, 1). His aspiration to create a national health service was predicated on his knowledge of how poorer communities could act collectively to enrich themselves through the combined effects of self-education, trade union membership and political organisation.

In his report, Beveridge famously identified the "five giant evils" of "want, disease, ignorance, squalor and idleness" (Beveridge, 1942). Like Bevan, he was clear on how health needed to be a policy priority at a time of collective exhaustion as the UK was recovering from the prolonged war effort. "Attack on disease is a matter of prevention; second of cure", he emphasised (Beveridge, 1942). The creation of the NHS can be seen as arising out of joint moral missions that emerged in the post-war period. This saw the liberation of British citizens from the evils of Nazism and fascist regimes abroad, by way of egalitarian policies enacted domestically. In so far as the former colonial territories were concerned, Bevan believed that peace "cannot be based permanently on colonial exploitation" (Bevan, 1958: 4). "Emancipated colonial peoples can rarely hope to continue to enjoy personal liberty as well as national independence unless some aid from outside is available", he argued. If Western nations wanted to see democracy extended, then they "must be prepared to compensate for the years of neglect and to underpin the political institutions of the new nations with part of their own wealth" (Bevan, 1958: 5).

Bevan brought a nuanced, if staunchly materialist, understanding of how to build a vision of the future out of the multiple devastations and losses brought about by the war. Churchill's stubborn character, though apt for wartime defence, was not a character trait that would enable the new victories or institutions needed the future, he argued: "what he did not do, and what he could not do, was to summon the future. For Mr Churchill is a spokesman of his class" (Bevan, 1940). Bevan was only in favour of what he called a "people's war" to the extent that it would lead to a new social order in peacetime. Following Britain's war victory, Bevan captured the new public mood through a question framed in temporal terms, a recognition that people could withstand suffering for a period, but not endlessly: "Why should the people wait any longer?" The concept of sacrifice would not hold, if not redeemed, contemporary researchers into the NHS acknowledge: "Sacrifices directly influenced post-war promises to build a new and better Britain" (Mohan & Harris, 2021).

Bevan chose to acknowledge the crucial role of the war in enabling the NHS to come into existence by way of quoting Karl Marx. "War passes supreme judgment upon social systems that have outlived their vitality" (Burtenshaw, 2019). His brand of parliamentary socialism was strongly informed by his understanding of class war. As the author of a recent thesis on Bevan's political thought affirms, Bevan adhered to "an orthodox Marxist understanding of social development that emphasised the centrality of the material base of society in determining its political and ideological structures" (Davies, 2019: i).

As Minister for Health between 1945 and 1951 he explicitly set out to create a health service whereby "the rich and the poor are treated alike," a system whereby "poverty is not a disability and wealth is not advantaged" (Bevan, 1952). This new service would ease the anxieties and fears felt by workers when unable to pay for healthcare, should illness arise. In his book, *In Place of Fear*, Bevan located health as "the field in which the claims of individual commercialism come into most immediate conflict with reputable notions of social values' (ibid, p. 53). He conflated good health with his own avowedly socialist concept of collective health, positing preventive medicine, as "merely another way of saying health by collective action", one which "builds up a system of social habits that constitute an indispensable part of what we mean by civilization" (ibid, p. 73).

AUSTERITY THEN AND NOW

Bevan's easy phrasing—"another way of saying"—attests to the mixture of "ideology and pragmatism" that allowed him to "win" the NHS it has been claimed (Broxton, 2017). He brought lived experience of poverty and inequality and an intuitive awareness of how social conditions act as determinants of health. Bevan understood that a rise in living standards was the best guarantee of health, an understanding gained not through empirical research since "this was not abstract question for us" (Bevan, 1948: 1).[12] Bevan declared that the NHS represented "what a socialist really means by socialism", considering it a "practical illustration" of the guiding Marxist principle "from each according to his capacity; to each according to his need" (Bevan, 1950: 14).

His vision for the NHS was not utopian but based on his experience of seeing a model work well at a local level. His successful effort to 'Tredegarize' the rest of the country was an act of faith grounded in experience, despite the fact that not all parts of country held dear to Tredegar's political values. This fact did not deter him. Rather, he described the NHS as "an attempt at the introduction of an egalitarian model through the medium of a society that is not egalitarian, either in its structure or inspiration" (Bevan, 1948: 7).

Such a belief stands in sharp contrast today to those who wish to limit the potency of Bevan's ideas by way of historical context. Indeed, some use this *same history* to show how things might have been done differently. Editors of a publication titled, *Devo-Then Devo-Now*, speculate on "what the history of the NHS can tell us about localism and devolution in health and care" (Quilter-Pinner & Gorsky, 2017). They note that "the marginalisation of local government (by Bevan) was not inevitable" (ibid, p. 2). "The history of health and care is an invaluable tool for policy makers today" because "there is often an implicit assumption that our existing system has been designed by logic and evidence alone, and therefore has some specific right to endure" (ibid, p. 5). They cite Bevan's argument in order to disinhibit constraint in re-shaping the NHS now, on terms that Bevan actively resisted then.

This research was commissioned by the IPPR, a think tank well-disposed towards the experiment of *Devo Manc* undertaken in Manchester in 2015. This new form of devolution marked the first occasion for NHS services to revert to local authority control since the NHS was created. Health and culture would further be combined through local Arts in Health policies adopted across Manchester's many boroughs, such as Oldham: "Not a forced association" but joint working arrangements enacted "intentionally, rather than leaving it to happy accident" (Higgins, 2016). Other researchers—those more sceptical of English regional devolution than the IPPR—queried the basis of this secret 'deal', seeing it as more as a financial "delegation" of austerity by central government, as much as the granting of autonomy to local government (Dorman et al., 2016: 3).

The economic 'logic' of George Osborne's policies of austerity was firmly rejected in a Lancet Commission dedicated to the topic of culture and health published in 2014. This sets the link between austerity and health within a longer historical and anthropological context. Other histories and places are claimed as marking the "origins" of the NHS here, "neither national nor English" (Napier et al., 2015: 1627).

The basic structure of the NHS was adopted in 1948 from a plan begun in Scotland in 1913 (and set out formally in 1936) to attend to the neglected health needs of rural poor in the Scottish Highlands and Islands. (ibid, p. 1627)

The Highland clearances are given as a reason for how "longstanding social collapse" in Scotland was a "brutal disaster" that forced "regional community health innovation" by necessity, not choice (ibid, p. 1628). A critical reading is given here of the punitive and corrosive effects of policies of austerity brought about through a deliberate desire to restructure systems of care in this way:

In times of great economic stress and societal change - as when governments implement strict austerity measures - trust can be paradoxically eroded through the very actions designed to enforce fiscal responsibility. (ibid, p. 1928)

It further states, rather presciently in retrospect, that:

Tolerance is rarely sustainable in insecure social settings where consensus, social agreement, and basic trust are put at risk. This decreased tolerance is evidenced not only in moments of extreme social suffering, such as wars and epidemics, but also when systems of health care are radically re-engineered, even in the interest of innovation. (ibid, p. 1627)

Forced innovation, brought about by fiscal restructuring, is condemned here as "wholly unacceptable" since the "moral costs" inflicted are too high (ibid, p. 1627)—with choices forced more through immiserating deliberation than happy accident. One voice based in Greater Manchester challenged Osborne's policy of austerity when compared to those deployed in the postwar years. The Director of *The North West Arts in Health Network*, Clive Parkinson, made the point that "When Britain was officially bankrupt... the government built its greatest public institutions" (Parkinson, 2011, 2012).

Parkinson refuted the claim that citizens can no longer afford a comprehensive health service, expressing the fear that Arts in Health might be reduced to the provision of "cultural quick-fixes for a fractured society" (ibid, 1). He named anxiety around Arts in Health interventions being adopted on this opportunistic basis since, he speculated, they could reflect a "morally-bankrupt society" as much as a financially sound one. Parkinson demanded a "fairer" not a "bigger" society (or smaller state), one that did not risk putting, as he portrayed it, "sticking plasters on infected wounds" (ibid, 2).

The limit of short-term repairs, enacted by way of inadequate 'patching', was also articulated by Beveridge, we can note, who saw how the scale of the destruction wrought by the Second World War as one that offered "opportunity for using experience in a clear field… A revolutionary moment in the world's history is a time for revolutions, not for patching" (Beveridge, 1942). This ambitious intention aimed to vanquish the slogans of austerity used in the Second World War, those which urged citizens to 'make do and mend'. Beavan demanded the wholesale re-thinking of the UK state apparatus, its social orientation, public value and institutional infrastructures—all at a time of national bankruptcy.

DESIGNS ON LIVING

The NHS was claimed as a "prized symbol" of Britain's "national status and Modernity" (Bivens, 2015: 13). Up until the establishment of the welfare state, experimental health centres in disadvantaged regions of London had pioneered holistic approaches to health and healthcare. First established in the 1930s, these tested how preventative health could be promoted in local communities, using architectures that deployed Modernist design principles. The built environment was itself conceived of as a therapeutic space, one able to facilitate social relationships and promote healthy behaviours. This understanding of architecture would find fuller expression in later decades when space was more fully understood as "intrinsically social, and social life intrinsically spatial" (Hillier and Hanson, 1984). Architectural design has always formed a part of the 'art' in Arts in Health, in this way, one more explicitly claimed as such in later decades (see Chapter Four).

The best known of these Modernist architectural examples is perhaps The Peckham Experiment, or Pioneer Health Centre, built in south London in 1935. This began as a research project intended to explore the causes, not of illness, but of health. It was conceived by two doctors (Scott

Williamson and Innes Pearse) who invited local families to join the centre for a subscription fee that allowed them to use this new facility for leisure and health. The bespoke design of the building encouraged behaviours through the adoption of new glass façades and movable walls whereby:

> The transparency of the building existed to allow surveillance by the doctors, but it was also said to embed an aesthetic of human activity that encouraged participation in the Centre's activities. (Zook, 2022: 8)

Central to its ethos—one underlined by its research methodology—was that people should be free to use the space as they wished. Otherwise, doctors would only serve as interference in their own research. Its day-to-day activities were organised through a committee with powers of self-governance. A sense of autonomy continues to be held as key to achieving good health, one that allows us to gain "a sense of coherence" over our lives (Antonovsky, 1979) and a "sense of control" over our environment (Marmot, 2010). Designed with this freedom in mind, "The building was accordingly open, flexible and programmed for self-directed and spontaneous activity" (Zook, 2022: 10).

Another example, albeit one conceived with a different intent, was the Finsbury Health Centre. Built in North London in 1938, architect Bernard Lubetkin based his design "on the aesthetics of our age," one intended to "convey the optimistic message of our time—the century of the common man" (see note 10). This institution came about as result of municipal efforts to improve the lives of the people living in this area driven by a local (South Asian) doctor, Dr Chuni Lal Katial. As chairman of the local authority public health committee, Katial wanted to centralise local services, seeing first-hand the disadvantage of piecemeal ad hoc developments. His was "an idealism rooted in the practical power of the local state to transform lives and raise the condition of the people" it has been subsequently claimed (Broughton, 2013). His achievement remains heralded today as "anticipating the foundation of the NHS by a clear decade", a symbol for "Modern healthy thinking and progress" (Allen, 2012) (Fig. 2.1).

A poster of the *Finsbury Health Centre*, created in the war year of 1943, presents a vision of a clean, bright, modernist medical facility for peacetime use in a near future. This is contrasted with the dilapidated state of a war-damaged Britain, one stained by 'disease'. Poor, sub-standard housing, exacerbated by wartime bombing, is highlighted in the depiction of

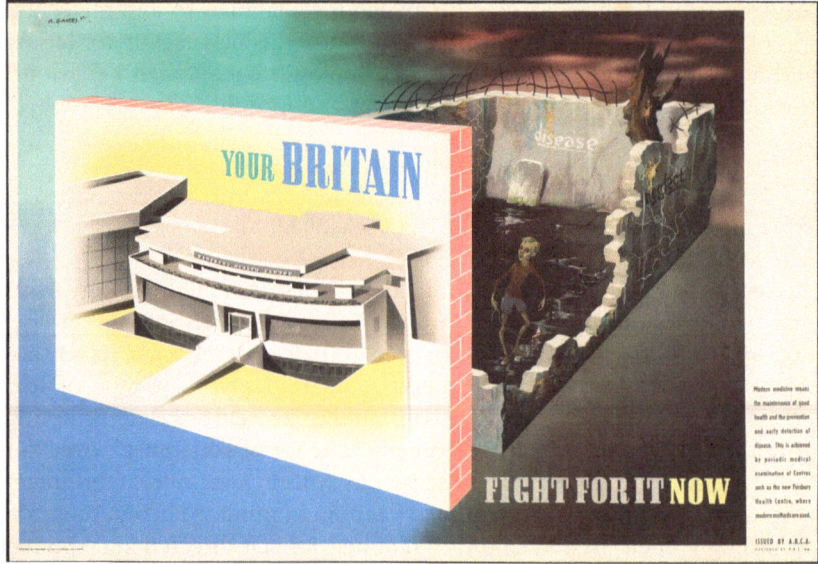

Fig. 2.1 The Finsbury Health Centre fronts a shared new vision for Britain set against the ruins of the war

derelict physical infrastructure.[13] Lubetkin believed that "nothing is too good for ordinary people" and using a metaphor of amplification, said he wanted his design to act as a "megaphone for health" (an arresting metaphor of the voice, or call to action, expressed through architectural form). Social justice on the Home Front is presented here as an extension of the fight against Fascist Nazism abroad: the encouragement offered on this poster is one which urges returning troops to continue to fight for '*Your Britain*'.

This sense of Britain belonging to all its citizens, and not just the country's ruling political elite, is one that would be played across rhetoric of both The Left and Right in subsequent decades. *Devo Then/Devo Now* authors describe how the 'NHS' acronym was first used in Labour Party "propaganda through political speeches given in the 1930s" (Bivens & Crane, 2017: 10). These three letters were chosen, they assert, to reflect the radical changes in medical provision that the new system represented, those intended to show the limitation of "variable and often unequal" services, with people "reliant on a patchwork of charitable, philanthropic and governmental funding" (ibid). Bevan's intention to 'Tredegarize' the UK was a prospect that set fear in the hearts of some right-wing newspaper editors of the period who characterised the move as a "tyrannical", even a fascist, threat:

> The State medical service is part of the Socialist plot to convert Great Britain into a National Socialist economy. The doctors' stand is the first effective revolt of the professional classes against Socialist tyranny. (*The Daily Sketch*, 1948)

Such conspiracy theories built on Winston Churchill's own damning characterisation of Aneurin Bevan as a "curse to his country in a time of peace". National character, as much as National survival, was seen to be at stake in the war years when Britain's integrity as a nation state was threatened by external forces and "all sources of comfort to our spirits were at a low ebb" (Kenyes, 1945). The military concept of 'morale', rather than that of 'well-being', was recognised as a crucial psychological aspect of the war effort, with 'culture' enlisted as an asset through the activities of two separate cultural bodies: the Entertainments National Service Association (ENSA) established in 1938 and the Council of Encouragement of Music and the Arts (CEMA) established in 1940. ENSA promoted variety performances and broadcast radio programmes for troops located across the world, keeping spirits up by way of comedy, tap, dance and song. CEMA's activities, by contrast, were focused on taking works of art from London out to the UK's regions and provinces, aiming to elevate humdrum lives. CEMA's would:

> carry music, drama and pictures to places which otherwise would be cut off from all contact with the masterpieces of happier days and times: to air-raid shelters, to war-time hostels, to factories, to mining villages. (Kenyes, 1945)

The economist Maynard Keynes took on the leadership of this CEMA in 1940 and made it a model for future cultural policy. Keynes proposed 'regional centres' were to be located around the country, as vehicles for his national vision for the arts in society. These would provide opportunity for the expression of cultural diversity:

how satisfactory it would be if different parts of this country would again walk their several ways as they once did and learn to develop something different from their neighbours and characteristic of themselves. (ibid)

Yet his choice of the CEMA model was also seen by many as "a lost opportunity", then as now (Williams, 1968; Hope, 2011). Keynes lent towards the democratising of culture (making high culture more accessible to working people) than adopting a route that promoted 'cultural democracy' (acknowledging existing working-class cultural forms and making the means of cultural production available to all). This preference continues to inflect cultural policy today with cultural democracy continuing to be championed as alternate model over many decades (Kelly, 1984; Jeffers and Moriarty, 2017; Leeson, 2017; Pritchard, 2017). Writing on Keynes' emphasis, the cultural theorist Raymond Williams locates this championing of high art as a sad loss, also seeing it as a failure of political judgement, too:

> The failure to fund the working-class movement culturally when the channels of popular education and popular culture were there in the forties became a key factor in the very quick disintegration of Labour's position in the fifties.

Bevan, we can note, held strong views of his own on the role of the artist in society in relation to its public funding. His vision for a healthy "civic life" was based on a belief that artists needed to be freed from the patronage of the wealthy few and serve the broader interests of society as a whole:

> Some day under the impulse of collective action, we shall enfranchise the artists, by giving them our public buildings to work upon… it is tiresome to listen to the diatribes of some modern art critics who bemoan the passing of the rich patron as though this must mean the decline of art whereas it could mean its emancipation, if the artists were restored to their proper relationship with civic life. (Bevan, 1952: 72)

This version of "emancipation" for arts would be more fully articulated by cultural critics writing in the 1950s and 60s, who would affirm a broader understanding of culture as 'a whole way of life' (Williams, 1959). Sociologists would challenge definition of The Arts as a luxury commodity acquired through 'good taste', framing culture as the very medium through which class distinction was felt and reproduced (Bourdieu, 1965). In his critique of the eponymous *Cambridge Tea Shop*, Raymond Williams found the "cultivated" tea drinkers here "not particularly learned", nor "practised in art", but those who nevertheless exhibited a sense of cultural entitlement based on class: "They had it and they showed you they had it" (Williams, 1959: 93). The French sociologist, Pierre Bourdieu, would go on to advance his concept of "habitus" to describe normative ways of thinking, feeling, acting and experiencing culture by members of social groups. "Social order is progressively inscribed in people's minds' in this way through 'cultural products'," (Bourdieu, 1984: 471).

Both Bourdieu's and Williams' analyses of culture are claimed as relevant to how creative health might be understood today, if fleetingly and discreetly, within the APPGAHW report.[14] "We adopt and broaden Pierre Bourdieu's designation of the 'cultural field' as the territory in which the arts engagement takes place" (APPGAHW, 2017: 10). Aneurin Bevan perhaps came the closest to arriving at Bourdieu's future description of habitus, when he said that public health relied on "a system of *social habits* that constitute an essential part of what we mean by civilisation" (Bevan, 1948, *my emphasis*). But in pinning his definition of culture so closely to 'civilisation', cultured (British) subjects are once again situated in opposition to those 'uncivilised' natures embodied by the colonial subject.

LOW MORALE, HIGH ART

This problematic framing of health and culture by way of 'civilisation' was perpetuated in the 'first steps' taken towards Arts Policy made by Jennie Lee (Lee, 1965). A fellow member of the Cabinet who was married to Nye Bevan, these two socialist politicians surely present the most manifest example of arts and health existing as "natural bedfellows" (to quote Mike White on this point). Lee would go on to publish the first ever White Paper for the Arts in 1965 which asserted that the "enjoyment of the arts should not be regarded as remote from everyday life" (ibid, p. 6). Rather, the "arts and (their) associated amenities should occupy a central place" in any 'civilised community', (ibid). These proposals were set amid a wider call for "a new social as well as artistic climate" yet to come, one whereby the country might become less "drab and joyless" and "more cultivated" (ibid, p. 19) (Fig. 2.2).

The heroism and dignity of healthcare workers was celebrated through art works created in the post-war years. The hospital drawings of Barbara

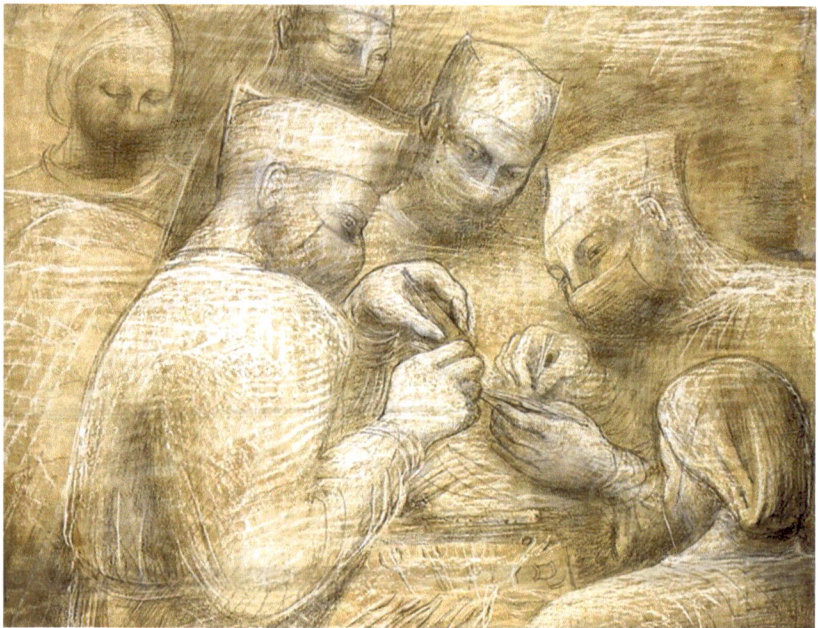

Fig. 2.2 One of Barbara Hepworth's Hospital drawings, in praise of collective action

Hepworth, for example, depict idealised surgeons at work in the operating theatre (1947–49). These were described as "works of socialist art" by one contemporary art critic in 2012 in that they "glow with a common purpose" and a "concentration on a shared task" (Jones, 2012). Jonathan Jones interprets the drawings as depictions of public virtue alien to our own age, one to which "austerity has returned" but without a belief in art's power to "save souls".[15] He quotes Hepworth directly in his review, to reveal her feeling towards her subject, one of intense admiration:

> From the moment when I entered the operating theatre I became completely absorbed by... the extraordinary beauty of purchase and coordination between human beings, all dedicated to the saving of life ... and the way that unity of idea and purpose dictated a perfection of concentration and movement. (Hepworth, 1970)

The Hospital Drawings offer alternative medical 'heroes' to the military heroes of the war, renditions that borrow visual motifs from angels depicted in Renaissance art. In passage from *In Place of Fear*, Bevan describes a very different kind of 'battle' in the operating theatre over that of any theatre of war. This is a class war, he asserts, not to be fought against foreign foes but figures of authority drawn from the ruling upper classes who show no concern for the lives of workers over whom they rule:

> powerful vested interests with profits at stake compel the public authorities to fight a sustained battle against the assumption that the pursuit of individual profit is the best way to serve the general good. (Bevan, 1952: 168)

He goes on to argue that the "same is true in relation to contagious diseases" since:

> These are kept at bay by the *constant war society is waging* in the form of collective action...It would be a fanatical supporter of the competitive society who asserted that the work done in the field of preventive medicine shows the enslavement of the individual to what has come to be described in the United States as 'statism' and is therefore to be deplored. (ibid)

This charge of "fanaticism" was aimed at all those who proposed 'socialised medicine' as it would go on to be called in America. Unlike Bevan, they saw the post-war (socialist) state as a threat to individual (creative) expression and freedom (Hayek, 1944). The economist and philosopher, Friedrich Hayek, believed that it was important to "decentralize power to reduce the absolute amount of power exercised by man over man" (Hayek, 1944: 41). "The competitive market system is the only system designed to minimise power" relative to those exerted by any totalitarian state (ibid). Hayek identified what was happening in Communist Russia as an example of the dangerous extent to which the state was able to dictate all aspects of the lives of its citizens. His theory of freedom rested on entirely different precept to that held by Bevan:

> From the fact that people are very different it follows that, if we treat them equally, the result must be inequality in their actual position, and that the only way to place them in an equal position would be to treat them differently. Equality before the law and material equality are therefore not only different but are in conflict with each other. (Hayek, 1960: 87)

The belief that the NHS represents the over-bearing embodiment of centralised state control has taken hold through such neoliberal philosophies, one which carries with it the idea of the NHS as a remote bureaucracy (Studdert, 2017). It was on this basis that Jeremy Hunt, while acting as The Secretary of State for Health in 2015, claimed that as a result of the way the NHS had been set up, all "health secretaries have to discover their 'inner Stalin'" (Hunt, 2015). This remark stands in contrast to Bevan's claim that "no danger of despotism arises" due to the way the NHS has been configured in relation to the welfare state, which he saw as agent of redistributive justice. Similarly, the economist John Maynard Keynes insisted that artists and arts organisations would be free to distinguish their own aims from that of the state: "to do it as far as possible by supporting others rather than by setting up state-run enterprises…co-operation with all, competition with none." He added: "the arts owe no vow of obedience" to the state (Keynes, 1945). The semi-independent body of *The Arts Council of Great Britain* was conceived as having an 'arms length' relationship to central government.

Although dismissed by Keynes and other liberal economists in the 1940s and 1950s, Hayek's ideas would exert greater influence in subsequent decades when neoliberal models of governance began to be adopted in the UK in the late 1970s and early 1980s. These decades saw the adoption of "a post-welfare state model of social order that celebrates unhindered markets as the most effective means of achieving economic growth and public welfare" (Bell & Green, 2016). The welfare state would be portrayed as the enemy of freedom with power needing to be 'devolved' to the citizen "in efforts to empower them to become self-governing, enterprising individuals" (Ayo, 2012: 103).

This is a rallying point that George Osborne amplified in his effort to 'shrink' the 'big state' by way of austerity implemented at a local level. "The people of Britain…these are the people we are fighting for" (Osborne, 2015). To introduce the idea of devolution in Greater Manchester in 2014, he appropriated a line from a speech made by Aneurin Bevan in 1945, using the phrase "we are the builders" over seven times. "We are the builders. And let me tell you who we are building for. The working people of Britain" (Osborne, 2015). He omitted a significant portion of Bevan's preceding sentence, skipping any mention of collective suffering or dreaming. His words provide revealing omissions. Osborne's insistence rested on his earlier—much queried—assertion that "We are all in this together" (Osborne, 2012). Osborne did not acknowledge Bevan by name, in what was described by one political commentator at this time as an act of "political looting" (D'Arcona, 2015).

These are some of the echoes of political discourse that reverberate particularly in Greater Manchester, a city where Bevan announced the 'birth' of the NHS in 1948, and where George Osborne announced Manchester as the place to "let the devolution revolution begin" (Osborne, 2015b). Health localism, and more latterly English devolution, then has proven an influential force in re-structuring the NHS. Such moves raise questions around the degree of autonomy that individuals—and local governmental alike—should be allowed in relation to the (central) state.[16] It is not without irony that the ambition, articulated by one contemporary Arts in Health advocate, to "make arts interventions national services within the NHS" (Joss, 2018) has been attempted by way of an accumulation of contracts won through competitive tender across different NHS systems and local areas across Wales and England.[17]

Local authority contexts, as we shall explore in the next two chapters, have played a vital role in the development of Arts in Health. Today, the prospective benefits of any Arts in Health project must compete with other cost-effective services now procured at this level of budgetary control and public accountability. This is far more complex system of accountabilities than the proverbial "sound of a bedpan" which Bevan said, if dropped in Tredegar, would "echo down corridors of power in Whitehall". Bevan deployed an aural metaphor to speak of how financial accounting and democratic accountability might combine.[18] It is amongst the tensions exerted between tiers of national and local government, that those comprising the field of Arts in *Health* would start to generate their own political pressure and strategies, through their own bespoke institutions.

Notes

1. I borrow Mark Fisher's idea of 'hauntology' here (Fisher, 2009) as I did for a photo-essay on the role played by the St Thomas' hospital as emblem of post-war utopian thinking and site of 'culture war' (Williams, 2020).
2. Aaron Antonovsky's concept of 'salutogenesis' is frequently cited by those working in Arts in Health, with health held out as a positive "counterpoint to pathogenesis", or the development of disease. (APPGAHW, 2017: 17).
3. Burn's words can be read in their own context, reflective of the tensions over political and financial control, felt at the time when Scottish independence was discussed as part of the 2014 referendum.

4. This was an impression reinforced as army and navy personnel supplemented the roles played by medical professions: helping administer vaccines and constructing 'The Nightingale' hospitals—temporary medical centres speedily set up across the country, named after the iconic nurse of The Crimean War.

5. 'Our NHS, A Hidden History'. https://www.bbc.co.uk/programmes/m000xwz6.

6. Boyle publicly reported in 2016 that then-Health Secretary, Jeremy Hunt, demanded that the NHS section be cut down, and that Boyle saved it only by threatening to resign and to take the volunteers whose contributions dominated the Opening Ceremony with him. https://www.independent.co.uk/news/uk/politics/danny-boyle-nhs-celebration-tories-london-2012-olympics-opening-ceremony-a7129186.html.

7. This comment was made by Nigel Lawson when he was Chancellor the Exchequer in the 1980s.

8. This is a refrain that has been picked up subsequently and further distorted. Anti-vaccine groups have used inflammatory hate speech to compare healthcare staff to doctors prosecuted at the Nuremberg Trials.

9. The words of arts in health activist, Steve Goslyn, quoted in my thesis (Williams, 2020: 206).

10. As detailed on the website, https://savefinsburyhealthcentre.wordpress.com/history/.

11. Quoted from a recorded talk: https://www.sochealth.co.uk/the-socialist-health-association/members/distinguished-members/julian-tudor-hart/.

12. Writing in the preface for *In Place of Fear* he makes this distinction in terms that Teresa May would echo to describe health inequality: namely as a "burning luminous mark of interrogation" (Bevan, 1952: 1). May described health inequality as a 'burning injustice' in 2017.

13. A contrast that drove Winston Churchill to try and ban the poster, saying it was a "disgraceful libel on the conditions prevailing in Great Britain before the war".

14. The title of Raymond Williams' 1958 essay *Culture is Ordinary*, in his book *Resources of Hope: Culture, Democracy, Socialism*, supplies the single reference to 'socialism' in the whole of the report, sunk deep in its footnotes.

15. The exhibition in Wakefield's new art gallery was timed to coincide with the 65th anniversary of the creation of the NHS.

16. Ultimate control of health in Greater Manchester resided with the health secretary. During the pandemic, however, this reverted to a centralised model, with local council left little role to play in public health messaging. https://www.theguardian.com/society/2020/may/05/private-covid-19-tracing-disaster-councils.

17. Joss' company, Aesop, was awarded 2.1 million to work with Swansea Health Board in 2017. The same years saw it run a similar 'Dance for Health' programme in Norwich, commissioned by the local CCG. https:// wahwn.cymru/knowledge-bank/dance-to-health-   and   https://www. danceeast.co.uk/news/dance-health-sessions-start-norfolk-january.

18. A famous proverbial saying attributed to Bevan. See this blog titled 'what Nye Bevan actually said': https://reestheskin.me/what-nye-bevan-actually-said/.

CHAPTER 3

Organisers, Survivors, Healers

The previous chapter detailed how the institutions of the British state set the overarching framework within which any consideration of the relationship between 'the arts' and 'health' in the UK can be brought into relation. The creation of the NHS was informed by Aneurin Bevan's understanding of preventative health as a goal best achieved through "collection action". He was able to formalise this (implicitly socialist) principle through the redistributive mechanisms of the welfare state, exploiting the opportunity presented by the landslide Labour victory of 1948. Social movements emerging in the 1960s and 70s also deployed collective action to achieve their aims, embracing health issues both directly and indirectly. These activities were organised informally, outside of parliamentary politics, working in parallel or *counter* to state institutions (including the NHS and Arts Council of Great Britain).

Common understandings of social movements of this time hold that they were more concerned with identity politics than the distribution of social or political goods and so were distinct from the organised Labour Movement. But such distinctions can also be seen as symptomatic of "structural transformations that produced new conflicts and new classes" at this time too (Della Porta & Diani, 2010: 52). As will become apparent through the following narrative, inter-linked social movements present

© The Author(s), under exclusive license to Springer Nature   49
Singapore Pte Ltd. 2023
F. Williams, *When Was Arts in Health?*,
https://doi.org/10.1007/978-981-19-3617-3_3

nuanced examples of how health demands were advanced through culture and the arts—not through any singular British culture but by way of international counter (and sub) cultures.

Black Power, Women's Liberation, the Peace and Green movements, psychiatry-system Survivor and Disability Rights movements (as self-described at this time) challenged forms of medical knowledge, its practice and systems. Campaigns centered on diverse "conflictual issues" (Tilly, 2004) with patient organisations affirming human rights from within the NHS, exerting a "quiet" influence "no less revolutionary" it has been claimed (Mold, 2013).[1] With greater awareness of citizen entitlement, patient-citizens were able to assert their right to "be treated as humans, not specimens" (Hodgson, 1963). The language of rights was "adopted both to formulate defensive claims - rights not to be intruded upon – and to advance demands - rights to various kinds of social provisions and resources" (Rose, 1985: 199). One critic of medical power, writing at the time, suggests that state institutions were put under increased scrutiny by post-war publics less deferential towards authority, those who saw unforeseen "costs" come into play:

> The optimism of the post-Second World War industrialised society has been characterized by a preoccupation with tracing the progress and achievements of its institutions, rather than their adequacy, their adverse effects of their social and economic cost. (Taylor, 1979: 2)

Social movements questioned whose interests the medical establishment served, seen to benefit "mainly itself, big business and government" (Taylor, 1979: 3). The conflictual issues they identified "cut across conventional distinctions between private and public spheres", it has been usefully noted, with "health produced by certain styles of scientific knowledge and certain ways of organising it" (Della Porta & Diani, 2010: 53). Health activisms were informed by scholarly critiques of medicine which have since been taken up by those promoting Arts in Health over the decades in a number of ways. Early Arts in Health protagonists staunchly aligned with those who identified the need to limit the power of the medical profession. They worked to expose the medical profession's (illegitimate) claim on financial resource as a result. But biomedical knowledge has also increasingly shaped how the arts are (under)valued, now strategically conceded as operating within what's been called the "hegemony of the clinic" (Broderick, 2011: 106).

CRITIQUES OF MEDICINE

Critiques of medicine grew at a time when the medical establishment was implicated in a wider set of harmful economic relations and cultural discourses, commonly termed "the medical-industrial complex" (Ehrenreich & Ehrenreich, 1978). Like Bevan, American health activists operating in the 1960s identified the profit motive as incompatible with the equitable provision and access to healthcare. "The American healthcare system is not in business for people's health", since health is judged a "low priority" by a nation "whose resources are committed to military and economic expansion" (ibid, p. 1). Allied to the Western projects of modernisation and globalisation, health and economic inequalities were reproduced through "medical imperialism" (Schreier & Berger, 1974: Illich, 1979). Healthcare was no longer seen as one of the few or only "benefits of European Imperialism", but a discourse that "produced sickness", entangled in a "deeper collusion" with global systems of capitalist economic extraction and racial injustice (Anderson, 1998: 523). Accounts of medicine as a force for good—whatever the cultural or economic context in which it was practised—faced fundamental challenge. Political economists pointed to how histories of medicine revealed the "colonial production of disease," with "the more literary of them analysing medicine and public health as technical discourses of colonialism" (ibid, p. 523).

Contemporary British historians of healthcare have also used the idea of medical imperialism, we can note, to specifically describe the invitation extended to workers from former British colonies to work for the NHS. They situate the UK's domestic reconstruction after the war as one that drew on imperial legacies and implicit racial discriminations (Bhambra, 2021; Bivens, 2015). The creation of the NHS did not resolve social inequalities, so much as provide the basis for ongoing struggles to continue in a domestic context since "Imperial power relations cast long shadows" (Bivens, 2015: 2).

As outlined in Chap. 1, the APPGAHW report of 2017 claims that "the culture of healthcare tends too much towards the technical-industrial" (APPGAHW, 2017: 5). In locating this claim in writings from this period, it is Ivan Illich who uses this term to talk about the medicalisation of human experience beyond what is appropriate, necessary or ethical:

> By transforming pain, illness, and death from a personal challenge into a *technical problem*, medical practice expropriates the potential of people to deal with their human condition in an autonomous way and becomes the source of a new kind of un-health. (Illich, 1979: 72 *my italics*)

Illich flipped the assumption that good health might be achieved through good medicine, famously asserting how "the medical establishment has become a major threat to health" (Illich, 1979: 2). He used evolutionary (rather than revolutionary) theory to argue for his own interpretation of health as "a process of adaptation. It designates the ability to adapt to changing environments, to growing up and ageing to healing when damaged" (Illich 1979: 57). This disinvestment in the value of medicine, one made in order to better define 'health', finds an echo in the APPGAHW report.[2] Here, a strikingly similar distinction is drawn:

> The UK healthcare system is largely geared-up to addressing acute situations in which health is compromised. This prompts distinctions between health and medicine, between health and healthcare provision. (APPGAHW, 2017: 16)

Other critiques of the medical establishment advanced in the 1970s make similar points to those of Illich but place a different emphasis. In *Medicine Out of Control* (1974), Richard Taylor takes issue with how medical professionals, rather than patients, control the provision of local healthcare services. He argues that social problems formulated in medical terms serve to "depoliticize" the social and economic conditions that lead to ill-health. As a result, "the value of medical science has been vastly over sold" since its "contribution to good health and declining mortality rates has been negligble" (Taylor, 1979: 2). Mortality rates improved over the last 150 years, it is argued here, not as a result of technical advances in medicine, but "improvements in general social conditions" (ibid, 3).

This idea had been first developed by a British doctor in the 1950s similarly struck by his colleagues lack of curiosity about the "causes of the diseases they were treating" (McKeown, 1976: 5). The role of medicine in reducing mortality death rates was questioned by Thomas McKeown who studied how standards of living determine health across different populations, over time. He considered how the needs of local communities might find expression and legitimacy relative to the central state's ability to redistribute resources on a more equitable basis.[3] "Not as dichotomous or opposing choices, but rather as essential complements to each other" (Cosgrove, 2002: 729).

Alongside these accounts of the shortcomings of medical systems—penned largely by doctors and priests—a contemporary historian identifies popular resistance to biomedical power arriving out of broader social movements.

Victoria Bates ascribes public distrust in medicine to it being "used without consideration of the human subject" (Bates et al., 2014: 10). She cites how the Second World War had ended with the dropping of atomic bombs on two Japanese cities, prompting anxiety around the unethical application of scientific knowledge. Peace movements grew to protest Britain's continuing global ambition as a nuclear power in the 1960s. The use of scientific knowledge for weapons of war is "crucial", she argues, "for understanding the emergence of the 'humanities in healthcare' as *a named entity*" (Bates et al., 2014: 11, *my italics*). Two "interwoven assumptions" underpinned the emergent field of the Medical Humanities; "the arts and humanities 'humanise', while simultaneously technology and medicine 'dehumanises'" (ibid). Medical education was held responsible for this "deficit", with a "dose of the humanities" prescribed for healthcare students to steer them towards humane practice (Fox, 1985: 334).

Different understandings of the human subject proved central to concepts of human agency developed at this time. In *The Birth of The Clinic* (1973), Michel Foucault wrote about the development of the medicine profession in France, positioning this genealogical enquiry carefully amongst other critiques of medicine: "not written in favour of one kind of medicine as against another kind of medicine, or against medicine and in favour of an absence of medicine" (Foucault, 1973: xix). Rather, he intended to compose a structural study that, as he explained his aim, "sets out to disentangle the conditions of its history from the density of discourse" (ibid, xix). Discourses thus produce subjectivities as much as any carceral institution—such as the prison or the asylum—he proposed, undermining the viability of any "sovereign subject". As one contemporary Foucault scholar working as a mental health researcher in the UK frames this shift in thinking:

> To analyse the relations between 'the self' and power, then, is not a matter of lamenting the ways in which our autonomy is suppressed by the state, but of investigating the ways in which subjectivity has become an essential object and target for certain strategies, tactics and procedures of regulation. (Rose, 1990: 3)

Foucault's work has been "criticised for diagnosing a type of power that leaves no space for resistance", a writer within critical health studies observes (Diedrich, 2016: 20). Certainly, new understandings of state power—or 'biopower'—were articulated by Foucault whereby nation states developed "numerous and diverse techniques for achieving the subjugations of bodies and the control of populations" (Foucault, 1976). But despite this emphasis on subjugation, scholars such as Diedrich continue to see Foucault's work as an "attempt to discern the conditions of possibility for the emergence of new forms of agency" (Diedrich, 2016: 20).

Rejecting the role of the intellectual as a leader of the uneducated masses, Foucault proposed that "intellectuals must learn from those most exposed to power", since "theory is one more tool" in forms of political resistance it has been suggested (Pickett, 1996: 453). Hybrid forms of knowledge could develop between theorists, practitioners and political activists. Critiques of medicine found popular cultural expression, for example, in the student uprisings in Paris in 1968.

'The Medicine of Capital'—or bourgeois medicine—was explicitly singled out as form of medical power injurious to workers. Artists working for *The Atelier Populaire* produced posters that attacked 'toxic' consumerism by way of images of the human body dismembered under violent stress. In one poster, the human subject appears in broken form, a puppet of capitalist reproduction. Workers are offered medical care on this cruel, instrumental basis, it was claimed. The image is certainly suggestive of the need to (re)configure the worker as human subject, one whose sense of agency depends on a rejection of use-value in order to regain any form of life (Fig. 3.1).

Events in Paris impacted directly on UK social movements (for health). In a book looking back at the community arts movement, a detailed account is given of how "ideas about art, culture, and education emerging from France in the 1960s were influential" in the UK (Jeffers, 2017: 9). Shared understandings between the French animation and British community arts movements claimed culture as "a process, not a product", urging "participation not consumption" (Hare, 1991). Yet European influences, such as these, are rarely acknowledged in Arts in Health histories. This is the case despite the contemporary claim that the field is a social movement that draws closely on others, now and in the past. Norma Daykin notes that "there has been a long history of artistic expression at the heart of resistance to oppression" (Daykin, 2019b: 11). Yet she gives no account or explanation of how "international movements addressing inequalities" might have informed British politics or culture, especially those that "challenge cultures of poverty" (ibid, p. 11). Rather, she gives three brief examples, over three historic periods, in one sentence.[4] This is

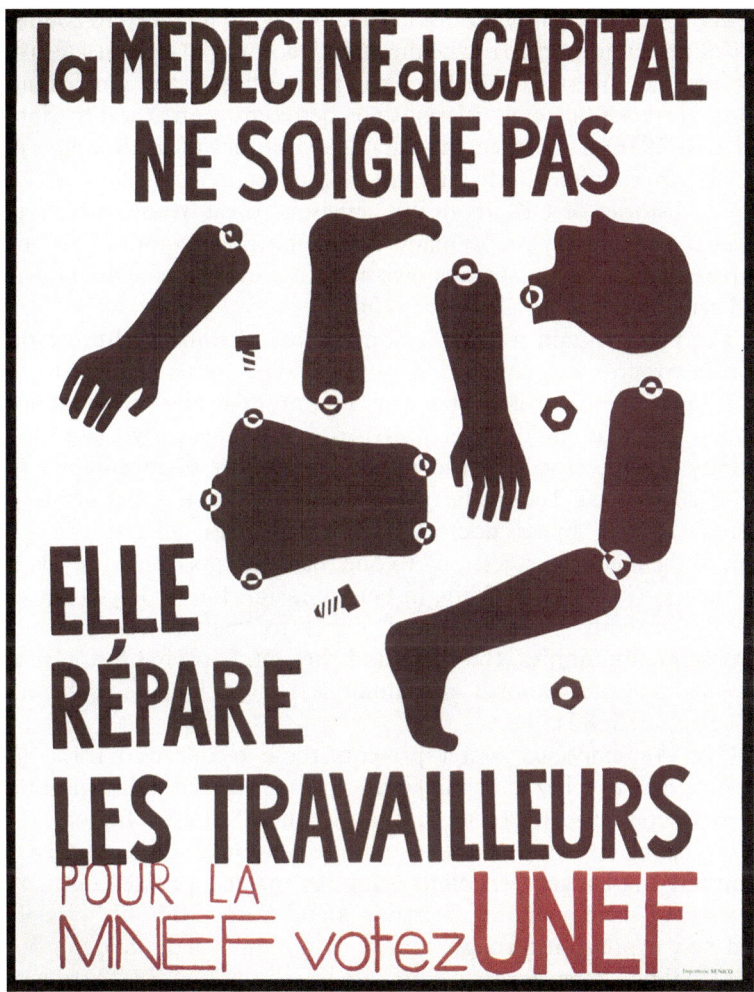

Fig. 3.1 'Bourgeois medicine does not heal. It repairs workers'

even more surprising, perhaps, given the prominence given to international perspectives in historical narratives which claim to chart the development of the field in Britain relative to the rest of the world (Clift & Camic, 2016).

The specific health activisms detailed below are intended to counter the risk of presenting a "narrowly internalist" account of Arts in Health, one that assumes "Western knowledge and perspectives… and simple unidirectional (or even bilateral) relationships between 'centre' and 'periphery'" (Bivens, 2015: 2). Rather, they draw on histories of medical knowledge which "are simultaneously international and idiosyncratically local" (ibid, p. 5). Histories of UK arts-health activisms reveal strong links to global social movements by way of many 'hidden histories' commonly motivated by patients' need to create their own narratives in the face of de-humanising and cruel 'treatments' (Diedrich, 2007).[5]

The personal and political commitments of some healthcare professionals towards the communities they served went beyond their allocated professional role. The case for "a new kind of doctor" was made—one that could play a more pro-active role as advocates for community health, especially the poorest and most disadvantaged (Hart, 1988). Welsh GP Tudor Hart, for example, suggested that primary care systems should "bypass doctors" altogether or else "change the orientation of the medical profession" to one that "accepts teamwork" as key to its success (ibid, p. 3). While in her campaign for sickle cell screening, nurse Elizabeth Anionwu found a way to "agitate for and mediate between communities, the NHS and the state", paying "explicit attention to the transnational communities to which patients belonged" (Bivens, 2015: 82).

One contemporary writer presents these reconceived roles, forged in the 1960s and 1970s, as marking a "haitus" in social relations, one that allowed counter-cultures to "invent wellness" afresh (Ingram, 2020). While failing to bring about revolutionary change at a structural level, Matthew Ingram argues, counter-cultures enabled a breach in the reproduction of social relations, hierarchies and norms. 'Health' was able to find new expression through culture, with new "methodologies of wellness" holding "transformative potentialities" (ibid, p. 7). These went far beyond "maximising of the individual's potential in a capitalist economy" or that of the "national state", he contends (ibid, 8). Proto Arts in Health initiatives ran separate, or in "parallel", to the healthcare cultures and structures of the state (Addae & Danquah, 2021), enacted through acts of "disaffiliation" as much as those of integration (Ingram, 2020: 1).

CROSSCURRENTS, UNDERCURRENTS

Mental health treatments represent, as seen in Daisy Fancourt's history, a point of ambivalence since "the arts were not always seen as positive for health" but could be seen as the cause illness through their indulgence in "excessive imagination" (Fancourt, 2017: 20). But beyond this negative framing, the "politics of madness" occupies a central, positive place in accounts of how the struggle to reconcieve and attain mental health was fought for in the post-war years (Robcis, 2021: 5).

'All power to the imagination' was the slogan chanted on the streets of the 1968 Paris uprisings. As Welsh cultural theorist, Raymond Williams, stated the value of the creative process: "Consciousness really does change, and new experience finds new interpretation: this is the permanent creative process" (Williams, 1962: 381).

One early radical re-imagination of mental health was developed at the Sant Alban Hospital in France by anarchist-doctor, Francois Tosquelles. Informed by his rejection of fascist ideology (he was forced to flee Catalonia in the 1930s), Tosquelles invited artists belonging to avant garde art movements (such as Dada and Surrealism) to take up place within the hospital. Here, within the scope of what he called 'institutional psychotherapy' (or *social therapie*), artists and the mentally ill shared a "similar goal: fighting against the 'absurd order' or the world" (Robcis, 2021: 35). Many others would go on to appropriate and valorise the 'art of the insane', as inspiration for movements such as *Art Brut*. Artwork produced by in-patients held in mental asylums was termed 'outsider art'—a phrase first coined by Roger Cardinal who curated *The Outsiders* exhibition, in London, in 1979.

Doctor-activists within the Tosquelles intellectual circle grounded their medical practice within older psychoanalytic traditions, believing that the psychiatric institution could act as a site of collective liberation if it were totally reconceived. Experimental new systems were staged both within and outside of the institution, a distinction itself thrown into question by psychiatrist, Franz Fanon. He interpreted the day clinic as an 'open door' institution, as site of productive exchange since:

> classical hospitalization considerably limits the patient's field of activity, prohibits all compensations, all movement, restrains him within the closed field of the hospital and condemns him to exercise his freedom in the unreal world of fantasy. (Fanon, 1960: 493)

Personal agency is only possible within the asylum in so much as it is enabled by a free society outside of it, Fanon suggests. The creation of experimental creative communities in France also took place in the UK, where art practice was pioneered as a therapeutic tool (as it was also in Italy and Germany).[6] The phrase 'art therapy' was first adopted in Britain in 1942 by Adrian Hill who proclaimed the foundational principle that "art can heal" (Hill, 1948: 30). Fellow pioneer of art therapy, Edward Adamson, likewise asserted art's role in "healing the mind", championing creative expression as therapeutic process (Adamson, 1984).

Individual creative expression was facilitated through group forums within institutional hospital settings in the 1950s, thought necessary to "create an atmosphere in which a journey of self-discovery could take place" (McNeilly, 1998: 114). Art Therapy went on to be championed in the UK as a clinical discipline practised outside the institutional context of the asylum but always under the overarching scope of the NHS—a process of legitimisation hard fought over for many decades (Hogan, 2001).[7]

More sceptical judgements of the institution as a potential site of healing would supersede the optimistic ideals informing *social therapie* in the late 1960s and 1970s. The creative re-invention of the mental health institution was no longer held able to enact any critique of power relations in society, so much as reproduce them. The "total institution" described by Irvin Goffman was, by contrast, "symbolized by the barrier to social intercourse with the outside that is built into the physical plant: locked doors, high walls..." (Goffman, 1961: 313). Those writing today, careful to distinguish between different types of institutional setting, point to how patients held within psychiatric institutions continue to experience "disconnection from pre-existing relationships and the imposition of a hierarchical social ordering whereby staff and residents occupy differentiated strata" (Series, 2021).

A key figure in UK antipsychiatry movement was Scottish psychiatrist, R.D. Laing. Intimate with the group of radicals at Saint Alban, Laing devised his own alternate psychosocial-therapeutic model at Kingsley Hall in East London. Doctors and patients lived together here at this site, adopting an informal arrangement where "no one had the right to give or receive orders, or to issue prescriptions. Kingsley Hall became a liberated parcel of land, a base for the counter-cultural movement" (Genosko, 1996: 46). Along with the British psychiatrist David Cooper, Laing acted as a popular catalyst for a re-evaluation of mental health services—and beyond that, society as a whole:

The anti-psychiatric critique rooted in a wider critique of society which, it was argued, is oppressive and requires the distortion and repression of human potentialities for its effective functioning. (Crossley, 1998: 878)

In this way, the "waves generated by this nucleus were powerful and wide-ranging," Nick Crossley contends (ibid, p. 880). "That Laing et al. inspired many 'patients' and young mental health practitioners is beyond question". Artists and other creatives are further credited as producing the "plays, films and paintings" that elicited wider public support and "pools of sympathizers" for victims of what was held to be an inhumane psychiatric system (ibid, p. 0). Other accounts of the relationships forged between Laing and his patients present a more problematic interpretation of his influence. While ostensibly disregarding forms of hierarchy, explicit hierarchies were reproduced on a more implicit basis, it's been argued (Genosko, 1996). Leading psychiatrists forgot "one of the elementary accomplishments of the first wave of psychiatric reform—that physicians speak to their patients" (ibid, p. 10).

Patients would go on to articulate their own experience of the UK mental health system on a more collective basis than the celebrity psychiatrists might allow. A manifesto written by *The Campaign Against Psychiatric Oppression* stated that "We have always believed that psychiatry cannot be reformed, so must be abolished". The Scottish Mental Patients Union was set up in 1971 (ahead of the London branch in 1974), leading to the formation of a national federation of anti-psychiatry groups. Pamphlets and zines circulated through these networks, with visual representation of psychiatric distress a powerful tool for naming, sharing and better understanding the nature of the harms inflicted by the psychiatric profession and punitive systems of 'care'.

Comics strips afforded a popular creative genre that did not need "to provide evidence, logic or argument", a contemporary observer notes. Rather, they appealed "to the collective experiential knowledge of the psychiatric survivor movement" (Spandler, 2020: 129). These D-I-Y artforms enabled 'knowledges from below' to find form. "Hierarchically inferior knowledges, knowledges that are below the required level of erudition of scientificity" (Foucault, 1997: 7). Such epistemologies were also championed by those in the Feminist movement who challenged the basis on which doctors assumed authority under the guise of scientific objectivity. The women's health movement encouraged women to explore their own bodies as sites of (self)knowledge that needed to be reclaimed from the de-humanising effect of the 'medical gaze' (Foucault, 1973), as well as the 'male gaze'—revealed as partial "ways of seeing" (Berger, 1972). Visual knowledges perform several functions at once, Helen Spandler suggests in a book chapter which explores how "psychiatric contention" can be usefully "crafted" (Spandler, 2020). Spandler quotes Audre Lorde to make the point that the cartoon art form allows survivors of the mental health system to become "available to themselves" (Lorde, 2017) since only then could "their critique become available to others" (Spandler, 2020: 131). Comics can "facilitate a complex visual layering of subjective and objective experiences, bridging the gap between clinical facts and personal perception"—it is argued by many who claim zines as a type of "graphic medicine" (Williams, 2015).

Within ongoing shifts in perception around the extent to which the institution could act as a site of healing power, the role of the creative imagination in envisioning forms of freedom continued to be a preoccupation for those in social movements. Various manifestos set out strategies that could be implemented through informal groups focused on a range of societal oppressions. "The starting point of our liberation must be to rid ourselves of the oppression which lies in the head of every one of us," the Gay Liberation Front (GLF) Manifesto proposed in 1971. "In order to survive, most of us have either knuckled under to pretend that no oppression exists and the result of this has been further to distort our heads" (ibid. p. 1).

Only through 'consciousness raising' groups, the GLF and others believed, could liberation come about—through experiential education undertaken within group forums: groups "in which we try to understand our oppression and learn new ways of thinking and behaving" (ibid, p. 2). Once becoming aware of "the gendered nature of our oppression", such insights would "inevitably bring us into conflict with the institutionalised sexism of this society" (ibid, p. 3). Such pedagogies were also projects of reclamation, those which challenged the ownership over bodies as claimed by either state or market. *Our Bodies, Ourselves* (1973) defined health as "a state defined by an elite," since "Woman do not have the necessary power to determine medical priorities; they are determined by corporate medical industry and academic research" (ibid, p. 3). This was a power of self-definition that artists were well placed to facilitate for themselves and others. The self-reflexive medium of photography, for example, allowed Jo Spence to narrate her treatment from breast cancer since it traded on the invitation "for others to look, judge and have power over her body and herself" (Bell, 2002).

Different social movements forged alliance, with patient-artists working across causes. "Challenging the psycho-pathologisation of homosexuality was a key focus of struggle for the gay liberation movement and a touchstone issue for the anti-psychiatry movement" too, it is usefully noted (Spandler & Carr, 2021). Perception of such overlaps would become the basis for more rigorous political articulations of the 'intersectional', both in theory and in practice in the 1980s (Crenshaw, 1991; Hooks, 1981). In this way, both individuals and groups could be better understood as "existing dynamically across multiple axes of identity" (Bridges et al., 2017: 180).[8]

Other examples of community health activism evidence how patients and healthcare workers were able to unite to reject the British State's discriminatory legal framework. Charting health activism in Brixton in the 1970s and 1980s, for example, contemporary researchers identify this specific south London district (and its active Black community) as one where activists worked to "improve their health *in parallel* to official health institutions" (Addae & Danquah, 2021: *my italics*). They took inspiration from The Black Panther movement in the USA, learning about self-run health clinics that could enable "greater local agency over health" (ibid, p. 1). In explaining the lack of attention these initiatives have received to date, these authors point to how such projects were "often regarded as being under-the-radar" since they operated within a "counterculture subaltern (public) sphere" (ibid, p. 1). Such initiatives arose out of "offstage discursive spaces" where anti-racist activism was generated out of shared cultures and first-hand experience of racial discrimination. Individuals could, in this way, serve as "agents of health", "albeit a healthcare quite different from that sanctioned or even supported by the state and medical institutions". These (sub)cultural activisms were not confined to the UK capital in London but also sprang up in other UK cities in the North—such as Bradford (through the establishment of the Transcultural Psychiatry Centre), as well as Liverpool and Manchester (Christie & Hill, 2003; Fernando, 2005).

Community health activisms also took place, we can also note, in rural as well as urban settings. One campaign mobilised around a form of discrimination informed by understandings of "internal colonialism" proposed at this time (Hechter, 1975).[9] On his appointment as a GP working in a Welsh-speaking area of North Wales in 1970, Dr Carl Clowes found his patients relieved to be able to speak to him in their first, and for some, only language. This, along the closure of the local quarry, prompted him to try and revive the health of the village of Llanaelhaern through setting up the UK's first community co-operative here in 1974. Yr Antur (The Venture) aimed to sustain the lives of villagers by way of combined initiatives, saving the local school from closure by the local authority and generating employment through traditional arts and crafts (a ceramic studio and knitwear business).

This project was part of a holistic drive for health undertaken at a local level, based on the premise that a "wider prescription" was needed in order to secure the Welsh language as a vital cultural component of this community's health. A revival in the villager's fortunes was enabled through the establishment of a Welsh language learning centre at nearby Nant Gwythern.[10] Yr Antur connected with the broader (Welsh) nationalist movement at this time led by groups such as *Cymdeithas Yr Iaith Gymraeg* (The Welsh Language Society) who self-describe themselves to this day as "a non-violent movement, part of an international revolutionary movement for rights and freedoms".[11]

The community health campaigns detailed above, then, in their different ways, challenged the basis by which 'British' identity was dictated by law or mispresented as a monoculture. While Yr Antur asserted the legal right to health equality on behalf of Welsh-speaking communities within the UK, Black British communities sought to re-define the status and entitlements afforded by Black British citizenship. Together they challenged what could fell under the scope of the British State through its exclusionary, discriminatory health systems.

WEEDS AND OTHER MISFITS

So far, in this chapter, we have seen how critiques of medicine were advanced in the 1960s and 1970s through social movements and how these relate to Arts in Health narratives today—with the arts uniquely able to articulate 'knowledges from below'. We have seen how UK movements for (mental) health were strongly informed by broader international social movements. More commonly, however, it is the UK's community arts movement that has been cited as the vehicle that led most directly to the creation of the field of Arts in Health.

In now turning to this specific movement, we can note that this too brings its own hidden history, one "undocumented and certainly under-discussed" (Jeffers, 2017: 4). Writing in 2008, Mike White most emphatically "traces the roots" of a "new alliance" between arts and health in the UK to the "community arts movement in the 1960s" (White, 2009: 13). This genealogy has been reinforced more recently by creative practitioners who were themselves active in the 1970s and 1980s (Leeson, 2017; Jeffers & Moriarty, 2017) as well as younger cultural workers and researchers keen to revive the emancipatory idea of 'cultural democracy' as a concern and cause today (Hope, 2011; Pritchard, 2020).

Clarifying his claim, White locates the community arts movement amongst "international currents of radical thinking that challenged the role of art in society and the aloof realm of commodified high art" (White, 2009: 13). Certainly, the art gallery and its 'white cube' had been made subject to rigorous critiques which cast this model as an exclusive reposi-tory of cultural capital and class privilege (O'Doherty, 1986). But this plac-ing of the community arts movement amongst "international currents" also blurs some of the distinction which can be made between its status as an 'art movement' and a 'social movement' or how it can be thought about as containing elements belonging to both. One artist writing at this time described it as the outcome of a semi-legitimate union: "The love child of alternative arts and community action" (Gregory, 1980: 20).

A central concern was to "give people access to the production of all forms of creative expression" (Jeffers, 2017: 4). Artists set up open stu-dios, photography labs, press and print workshops—technologies of reproduction still out of the reach of most people in this pre-internet period. Community artists sought to make it possible for everyone to take up their 'right to make art' wherever they lived (Jeffers & Moriarty, 2017) recognising a need to "decentralise cultural resources, production and dis-tribution" away from London (Leeson, 2017: 5). Community artists worked across all regions of the UK in a bid to facilitate 'cultural plurality'. It was hoped that different communities, especially those considered 'mar-ginal', might become more actively engaged in political and democratic processes as a result:

> Some artists reacted to the perceived injustice of the situation where many people had little opportunity to practise the arts due to a lack of resources and opportunity imposed on them by unequal distributions of social and cultural capital. Some artists had a political project in mind. (Jeffers, 2017:1)

A focus on creative means, over ends, produced "a *new* kind of political activist who believed that creativity was an essential tool in *any* kind of radical struggle" (Kelly, 1984: 12 *my emphasis*). Artist Lorraine Leeson grants us insight into this new role for the artist in an account she gives of her working practice from this time. Along with Peter Dunn she was commissioned through a local authority scheme—The Greater London Arts Fellowship—to set up film and video workshops in East London in 1977. Premises for their workshop were made available through a social worker involved in the campaign to save Bethnal Green hospital, with links forged between the artists and the campaign committee over time (Fig. 3.2).

One didactic montage juxtaposes image and text and invites the viewer to choose between an acceptance of "their economics" alongside the choice to protect "your health". These possessive pronouns perhaps hide the more nuanced entitlement to interpretation which informed the artists' brief—one which saw her tasked with conveying a political point beyond that of her own interpretation alone. While "producing the work ourselves", Leeson says that she referred "to the campaign committee regarding the meanings to be portrayed" (ibid). This was in line with an

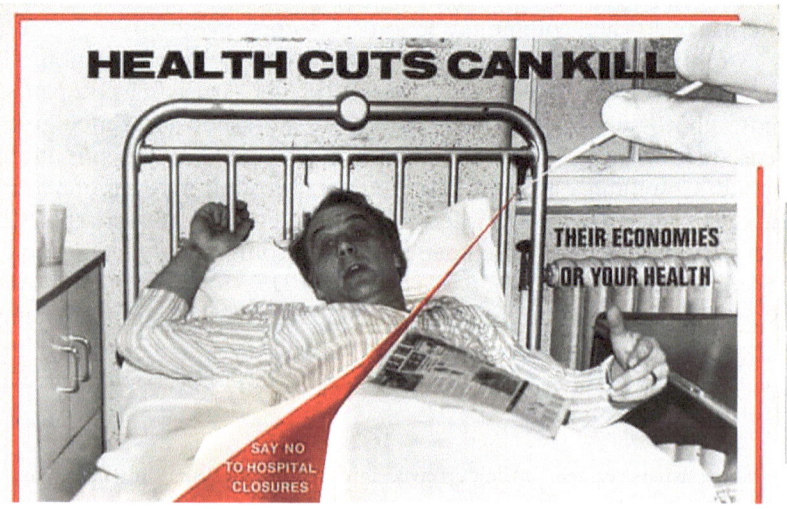

Fig. 3.2 Lorraine Leeson's poster produced as part of the campaign to save Bethnal Green Hospital, 1978

ethos that placed the community artist more as an "enabler or animator" than the sole figure able to make decisions pertaining to art production (Gregory, 1980: 20).

The choices enabled by certain economic rationales would go on to become a central contention for those working out of the community arts movement who campaigned for their activities to be funded by both local and national funding bodies. While local authorities proved receptive to artists embarking on collective endeavours, such as Leeson (she went on to work as an advisor to the Greater London Council), the Arts Council of Great Britain (ACGB) continued to be identified as a block to progress, an "obstacle to achieving the kind of democratic and equitable access to the means of cultural production" (Kelly, 1984: 49).

Orientated against this state-funded body, artists involved in the community arts movement portrayed themselves as illicit interlopers, "dandelions" taking root in places that the cultivators of Great British culture refused to sanction. This choice of wording was used in response to an earlier policy document titled, *The Glory of the Garden*, published in 1951 which had urged the Arts Council of Great Britain to discriminate on the basis of quality: "few, but roses" (Harvie, 2013: 18). Indeed, the dandelion metaphor informed a direct action outside of the offices of ACGB offices in 1975 when artists carried placards which:

> fitted together to create a giant image. On one side, there was a profusion of golden dandelions surrounding a single rose, dripping poison and covered in thorns. On the other side a slogan read 'Never Mind the Roses, Fund the Dandelions'. (Moriarty, 2017: 68)

This image of misplaced investment must be seen as part of a broader campaign to expand the types of art forms funded by the ACGB at this time. A total re-conception of the arts and culture was taking place, one which championed the 'ordinary' over the elitist (Williams, 1972) as well as the avowedly 'experimental'. *The New Activities Committee* (1968–1970) was set up to consider applications beyond those utilising accepted mediums, with 'community arts' set alongside 'performance art' within a newly formed *Experimental Projects Committee* (1970–1973). The receptive conditions afforded to new forms of art informed another artist group that emerged, namely *The Artist Placement Group* (APG). Like the community arts movement, this too has been claimed as an important strand of arts practice that allowed us to "rethink the artist's role in society" (Bishop, 2010: 163).

The APG rejected direct action in favour of more idiosyncratic and integrative strategies, with time and space a central preoccupation of their conceptual, durational, process-based work. Artists were placed in institutions for indefinite periods and aimed to open up new ways of thinking through becoming co-workers. "An artist would enter an exclusive environment of power and interact with employees at all levels of the institution, from management to shop floor" (Bishop, 2010:1). Between 1966 and 1980, the APG negotiated fifteen 'placements', some with industrial corporations (such as British Steel and ICI), others with governmental departments including the Department of Health and Social Security.

Artists would work to an open brief: "the status of the artist within organisations is independent, bound by the invitation, rather than by any instruction from authority within the organisation". The hospital became a setting that Latham chose to focus after he was admitted to Clare hospital following a car accident in 1968. He used the X-rays documenting his convalescence to claim that he had discovered a way to improve medical procedures. Together with his crashed car, they formed part of an exhibition titled *inn7o* at the Hayward Gallery, an exhibition which explores diverse examples of "knowledge exchange" between artists and institutions. APG's artworks at this show exhibited, according to one of their peers, the "dramatic confrontation between artistic and corporate cultures" that were developing at this time (Leggett, 2012).[12]

This sense of building confrontation is perhaps better exemplified by another APG hospital placement which saw the artist Ian Breakwell work at the high-security psychiatric hospital at Broadmoor. Working alongside a team of specialists tasked with improving conditions for inmates, his multimedia journal was used by this team to introduce a "more consultative approach to their research, in which patients were asked for their views on the prison hospital" (Bishop, 2010: 1). The results "angered Broadmoor's administrators, who felt that the team had overstepped its brief and had 'embarrassed the higher level of the DHSS hierarchy' and consequently the research was—and remains—restricted by the Official Secrets Act" (ibid, p. 2).

Alongside Latham's adoption of the hospital for an impromptu placement of his own invention—and Breakwell's thwarted consultation—other artists sought to find a place for themselves within the hospital's hierarchies by covert means. Painter Peter Senior's approach aligned with the community arts movements aims to facilitate lay creativity from the bottom-up.

Working as a volunteer at St Mary's hospital in Manchester, he gained permission to hang his abstract paintings on the walls. This enabled him to canvas staff opinions on further design 'improvements', a quisling role that resulting in him being regarded as 'the hospital artist', he recounts (Senior & Croall, 1995: 9). This (false) perception of his institutional authority provided him with a "valuable passport" that allowed him to gain access the "whole of the hospital" while not "fitting into the organisational hierarchy" (ibid, p. 9).

Senior gives an account of what he calls the "birth of a movement" in a book he co-wrote with Jonathan Croall in 1993, titled *Helping to Heal*. The Manchester Hospital Arts project he established in 1974 saw four artists employed through the *Manpower Services Commission's Job Creation Programme*. Brian Chapman joined the team in 1976 to "explore alternative roles for the arts and artists within healthcare", a project of diversification which would evolve into the renowned hospital arts organisation, LIME. The basis for LIME's work was based on a holistic vision in line with a medical humanities approach: to "cure the whole person rather than just deal with their physical symptoms" (Senior & Croall, 1995: 93).

In parallel to Senior's development of a Manchester-based hub for different types of arts activities within hospital settings, national organisations began to forge exchanges through allowing artworks from their collections to find new homes in hospitals. The newly built St Thomas' Hospital in London was granted artworks on permanent loan from the nearby Tate Gallery in 1976. Moving beyond these ad hoc arrangements—forged by interested individuals rather than by way of any concerted design—strategic opportunities began to present themselves. Cross-sector partnerships were forged between various trusts and local authorities around the UK. The Kings Fund and Greater London Arts (GLA) joined forces to set up the Arts in Hospital scheme in 1979.

Regional arts councils outside of London would go on to support arts commissions within hospitals such as Brigit Riley's re-working of a corridor at the Royal Liverpool Hospital in 1987. Such transfers of context from gallery to hospital had to negotiate the relative monetary and social values ascribed to works of art re-sited in this way. While new benefits were enabled by the inclusive social spaces of the NHS, the transfer of work by a commercially successful artist—such as Riley—served to throw these mutually dependent social and economic contexts open to question.[13]

Victories and Defeats

As a result of support won from various funders, not just the state but trusts and foundations such as The Gulbenkian and Esme Fairburn, some within community arts movement saw art's critical capacities put at risk by "grant dependency" (Kelly, 1984: 155). Pragmatism had led the community arts movement to "seek money wherever it could find it and to imagine that this money came without any strings attached" (ibid, 14). Owen Kelly lamented what he saw as art activities which had become "one more branch of whatever the state choses to leave the Welfare state", with artists allocated roles as "kindly folk who do good without ever causing trouble" (Kelly, 1984: 12). In *Storming the Citadel,* he gives a searing critique of how "the community arts movement had no clear understanding of its own history, neither documented it… nor drawing any conclusions from it" (ibid, p. 13). While winning "real victories", this meant it could not predict future crisis, having no tools or capacity to "circumvent them" (ibid, p. 14).

Offering a longer (Welsh) retrospective view on the rise and fall of community arts, Nick Clements writes of working in the late 1970s when the movement's "pioneering spirit" was "commodified" (Clements, 2017: 103). He observed class differences, those that saw art-school trained practitioners take on the role of enablers to communities deemed in need of their services, but who were not always part of them. He writes how:

> as community artists we were witness to the Miner's Strike. None of us were miners. And it became very alluring to represent a voice opposing oppression when you really had nothing to lose. (ibid, p.103)

Clements upholds Kelly's point that the state "appropriated the very art that was meant to 'storm the citadels'" (ibid, p. 103), citing funding systems as the key mechanism by which artists were disarmed of their autonomy. While there used to be an "understanding you did such work for no pay, out of solidarity with the people you supported", the nature of solidarity changed when artists came with a fee. The "professionalization of the work inevitably led" to funders "asserting control" (ibid, p. 107). The term, 'Arts in Health', finds a specific mention at the end of his narrative, a point at which it finds expression amongst the "multitude of new names for the art being produced" in the late 1980s and early 1990s (ibid, 108).

Kelly's sense of impending crisis was confirmed by the election of Margaret Thatcher as PM in 1979, a watershed moment which marked a significant change in direction of government policy across all areas—especially that of public health. The Black Report presents a case in point, one that would deeply inform future developments in the emergent field of Arts in Health. This review of national health had been commissioned by the former Labour Secretary of State in 1977 but was published just after the new government assumed power in 1980. Its evidence showed that class difference was strongly reflected in health outcomes, widening not contracting despite the achievements of the NHS in the post-war decades.

Researchers such as Richard Wilkinson and Michael Marmot began to build on Thomas McKeown's earlier findings into the health of populations over time. They would go on to further investigate differences in mortality rates in the UK with much higher death rates lower down the social scale—reflective of the fundamental inequalities in purchasing power in our society. Setting out ambitious plans to address widening "health divides", *The Black Report* was notoriously supressed by the incoming government (it was published on a bank holiday) and its findings firmly rejected on the basis they were economically "unrealistic". While the political timing of the report could not have been worse, it was noted that the manner of its reception provoked "a kind of *underground culture* of inequalities research and debate which continued throughout the 80s and early 90s" (Berridge, 1999).[14]

Industrial policy and growing social inequality would go on to provoke further social unrest and industrial action, culminating in the National Union of mineworks strike of 1984. Using the language of subversion (much as tabloid newspapers had done in the 1930s) Margaret Thatcher questioned the loyalty of mine workers to the British State, notoriously calling them "the enemy within" (Thatcher, 1984). Monetarist economic policy was the catalyst for unlikely solidarities forged in the face of a common threat—which Thatcher herself came to represent and embody for many on The New Left. Campaigning groups such as *Lesbians and Gay Men Support the Miners* (LGSM) worked to build supportive links between all those opposed to Thatcher's ideological position mobilising across class and identity politics. LGSM raised hardship funds between support groups 'twinned' across mining communities and others spread across England, Scotland and Wales.

A postcard designed at this time uses the iconographies of socialist trade union solidarity to combine them with those of new wave social movements, including feminist organisers: a banner is depicted that reads 'Women Against Pit Closures'. Thatcher is portrayed as the puppet master of the judiciary whose anti-trade union laws were used to stymie the effectiveness of the NUM 'flying' pickets (those which saw miners travel from one area of the country to another). Such alliances were cast as a 'rainbow coalition', as presidential candidate, Jesse Jackson, termed them as part of his campaign (Jackson, 1984) But in this instance they reflected solidarities forged across industrial geographies and urban populations within the UK too (Fig. 3.3).

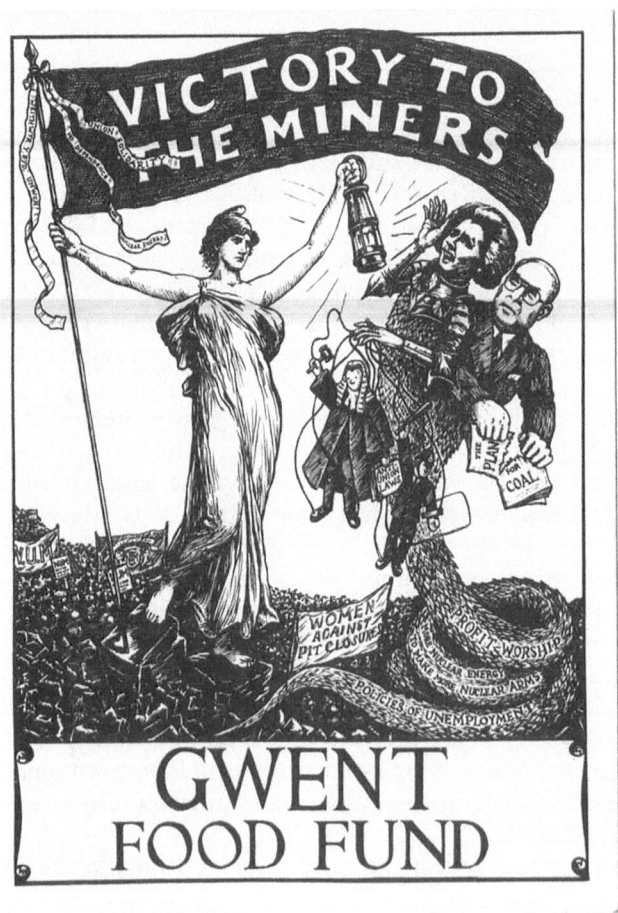

Fig. 3.3   Postcard produced by in Stoke Newington, London, in support of South Wales miners

LGSM marked a concerted response to a government that cast both these groups as disloyal 'outsiders', harmful to the body politic. The effect of stigmatisation was felt powerfully by gay men who at this time were dying in huge number from the AIDS virus—an epidemic dubbed the 'gay plague' in the tabloid press. The disease and its many impacts profoundly influenced how community organising and health activisms unfolded. The AIDS Memorial Quilt is cited in one of the first anthologies to name area of work *The Healing Arts* (Haldane & Loppert, 1999). This term was applied to harms caused not only by illness, but those exacerbated by political inaction and neglect and social stigma too. A tension is named in this book between the active "consciousness raising component" that the Memorial Quilt sought to provoke, alongside the more ameliorative aim to create "a healing narrative" through grief (Blumberg, 1999: 65).

Social inequality would deepen as a result of policies that saw the closure of heavy manufacturing in areas of the UK (in the North East, South Wales and Scotland). Unemployment soared to over six million, with riots breaking out across many cities in the UK in the early 1980s.[15] Black and minority ethnic communities were concentrated in these areas and, in response, health activisms intensified. The Liverpool Black Sisters began a campaign to "challenge the local council, health authority and local mental health officials regarding the racism that Black survivors of the mental health system experienced" (Wainwright & McKeown, 2019). They met with elected officials to demand that the local authority provide resource for respite and drop-in services, engaging in "protracted tense and at times emotional negotiations with the local council and health services" (ibid, 8).[16]

The Health and Race Action Research project, set up in Liverpool in the 1980s, would lead to the establishment of the Mary Seacole Centre (in 1991). In this way, local authorities provided the local democratic forums through which changes in local health services could be demanded and met. As contemporary chroniclers assert:

> From the late 1970s many radicals shaped by the New Left entered into the state and – as the central government began to defund local authorities – were on the frontline of a battle between central and local government that raged throughout the 1980s. (Davies et al., 2022:206)

The most iconic example was presented by the Greater London Council (GLC) which funded numerous arts projects that sought to promote equality and health. Sunil Gupta's 1986 exhibition *The Black Experience* was, for example, among the first to use public funds to photograph portraits of the lives of Black lesbians and gay men. The 1982 film *Framed Youth: Revenge of the Teenage Perverts* similarly challenged negative stereotypes, giving future artists a platform for early self-reflexive experiments in the new medium of video (Isaac Julian, amongst others).

"We will use expenditure on the Arts not to provide the icing on the cake, but as a part of the political ingredient of that cake…" was how Tony Banks, Chair of the Arts and Recreation Committee, framed his mission (in what proved to be his final term in office).[17] The GLC was abolished by Margaret Thatcher's government in 1986 after being made subject to attack in the popular press as 'looney left'. The (New) Labour Party did not come to the defence of regional local authorities pejoratively labelled in this way, but famously "joined in the denigration" (Panich & Leys, 2001: 217) with Neil Kinnock denouncing Liverpool's council in 1984.

Thatcher ascribed social unrest not to socioeconomic inequalities or class division, but personal inadequacy. Cabinet minutes recently made public from this period prove illuminating in relation to how the arts were rejected as a potential healing balm in this period of strife and social conflict. The Prime Minister was warned against setting up a £10 million pound communities programme to tackle inner-city problems by cabinet colleagues as it would do little more than "subsidise Rastafarian arts and crafts workshops" (Letwin, 1984). This racist characterisation rejects the use of culture as agent of social cohesion as much as it, perhaps, acknowledges the power of this potential too.[18] Proposals were made by Thatcher's government that they should simply "let Liverpool decline", a policy of strategic abandonment that would have seen people living in poorer areas neglected in order for wealthier ones to thrive. This policy—one that in effect explicitly promoted inequality—came close to rendering certain inner cities as no-go areas. It would have been a political choice that would have further absolved the need for central government to take measures to relieve the poverty of people living in these places.

In the event, a more interventionist approach won the day amongst her Cabinet, one whereby the figure of the entrepreneur would "breathe new life into Merseyside and Britain's other declining post-industrial metropolitan cities". In his report, *It Took A Riot*, Michael Heseltine countered the logic of abandonment as he thought it was "not compatible with the traditions of social justice and national even-handedness on which our Party prides itself" (Heseltine, 1981). His One Nation Tory approach was used to justify the encouragement of private enterprise as replacement for the (local) state.

Former industrial cities in the UK began to embark on what would become known as 'regeneration' processes. The power of the creative imagination would also be re-fashioned through a concomitant "gentrification of the mind", one LGBTQ activist has argued (Schulman, 2013). Speaking on what makes cities vibrant places to live, Sarah Schulman argues that "many languages, many cultures, many racial and class experiences take place on the same block". But with gentrification, "homogenous neighbourhoods erase this dynamic and are much more vulnerable to enforcement of conformity" (ibid, 36). These new city environments proved harder ones for sub- and counter-cultural groups to occupy—as former squats were claimed by property developers. Financialised capital would be ploughed into formerly 'edgy' inner city areas where artists once rented cheap studio space. A new approach—to poverty, place and health inequality—would take on greater momentum in the next decade, one in which the nascent movement of Arts in Health would find its own creative method and moral justification, one enabled through a newly re-structured national formation of its own.[19]

NOTES

1. Helen Hodgson set up *The Patient Rights Organisation* in 1963 demanding patients right to knowledge and consent to medical treatment, especially if part of a medical trial. This organisation "did not represent the interests of any one particular group of patients, but rather of all patients" (Mold, 2013: 226). More individual-orientated and market-based models of healthcare were adopted in the UK resulting in "individual patient choice appearing to edge out collective patient voice" (Ibid, p. 238).
2. Illich finds no direct reference in the report, though a quote provided by Iona Heath (an inquiry interviewee) is quoted making points that amplify his viewpoint: "The whole discipline of medicine has colluded in the wider societal project of seeking technical solutions to the existential problems posed by distress" (APPGAHW, 2017: 142).
3. McKeown's work has been "used as a way of containing costs and providing a rationale for doing so, without at the same time sharing the concern of the author for humane and equitable care" (Colgrove, 2002) That his ideas were used to justify UK government spending cuts was a "sad irony"

according to one reader, who laments the fact that his insights, though correctly surmised, were misapplied (ibid).

4. "From the Mexicanidad Movement of the 1930 featuring artists such as Deigo Rivera and Frieda Kahlo, the underground jazz scene in Nazi Germany and the oppositional role of rap and hip hop in African American popular culture in the 1990s" (ibid, p. 11).

5. Lisa Diedrich plays on words in her book title *Treatments* (2007) to talk about illness as an event that reflects wider cultural contexts.

6. The Socialist Patients Collective also operated in Germany and Franco Basaglia's movement for 'Psichiatria Democratica', in Italy.

7. In the forward to one history of Art Therapy, this profession is located 'in a history of psychiatry' (Hogan, 2001:10). Yet "it would be equally valid to argue that the story of art therapy belongs to a history of anti-psychiatry" (ibid p. 10). Such an ambivalence presents a provocation, David Lomas argues, around "how far art therapy's radical credentials are compromised" by this move (Hogan, 2001: 12).

8. Critical Race Theory, first developed in the late 1980s, would go on to acknowledge how individuals and social groups 'exist dynamically across multiple axes of identity', limiting essentialist readings whereby 'social categories such as "Black," "woman," and "disabled" are used to capture the totality of a person's health status without appreciating how these and other social, economic, and political positionalities intersect to shape health outcomes' (Bridges et al., 2017: 180).

9. This Dr Carl Clowes credited this 1972 book as one that informed his own understanding of the role of Wales in the creation of the British State. Others have since taken up this comparison (Price, 2016); questioned it as dubious (Johnes, 2019) as well as seeing it as 'beside the point' (Evans et al., 2021).

10. At nearby Nant Gwythern, a deserted quarry settlement brought back to life. See Nant Gwetheryn's website: https://nantgwrtheyrn.org

11. Acts of civil disobedience, inspired by the US civil rights movement, helped bring about changes in UK law to win equal legal status of the Welsh language (in 1993). Clowes steered the first Welsh language strategy that led to the Welsh Language Act, being passed. The creation of a Welsh-language television channel, for example, was a key demand alongside others for Welsh-language education and affordable homes.

12. Despite the APG "scrupulously avoided taking an oppositional stance toward the companies with which it negotiated" the government withdrew public funding on the basis that they believed that the group was concerned more with "social engineering" than with "straight art" (Bishop, 2010). Clare Bishop gives a nuanced reading of Latham's political neutrality in the face of criticism by Marxist critics in her review of the APG in *Art Forum* in 2010.

13. While being "delighted" by the commission, Riley notes that her work did "not have quite the same objectives as my other wall works" and makes her intention clear "not to interfere with the essential activities of the hospital", providing an "undemanding presence" against which the drama of life-saving interventions could be foregrounded. See https://fadmagazine.com/2014/04/03/art-news-stunning-56-metre-mural-by-bridget-riley-transforms-st-marys-hospital-london/

14. See this account of The Black Report's reception: https://www.sochealth.co.uk/national-health-service/public-health-and-wellbeing/poverty-and-inequality/the-black-report-1980/the-origin-of-the-black-report/interpreting-the-black-report/

15. Toxteth in Liverpool, in 1981, Brixton and Tottenham in London, in 1985.

16. It remains the only agency working with Black and Asian communities in Liverpool to this day, since other BAME agencies that emerged at this time were forced to close due to "austerity measures" that "threatened the few alternative mental health services". (Wainright and McKeown, 2019)

17. Thatcher claimed that such a London-wide authority was inefficient and scaled-down government to borough level. Wider discussion of why the GLC was abolished, and the role of local cultural policy in prompting this move is given by Brenden O'Leary, in *Why Was the GLC Abolished?* (2009).

18. Racist overtones that Oliver Letwin was forced to apologise for when he went on to also work for David Cameron in 2015, a time when this collection of private memos was declassified and made public. https://www.theguardian.com/politics/2015/dec/30/oliver-letwin-blocked-help-for-black-youth-after-1985-riots

19. Rather, the unemployed were urged to 'get on a bike' to search for work in other more affluent areas of the country as Norman Tebbit scolded, recounting his own father's strategy to gain employment in the 1930s.

CHAPTER 4

Missionaries, Parasites, Mitigators

In the last chapter, health activism in the UK in the 1960 and 70s was shown to have been informed by international social justice movements, with counter (and sub) cultures the vehicle for health activisms. Novel social solidarities between artists, patients and doctors were forged that allowed discriminatory practices and professional hierarchies to be re-imagined and breached. But the capacity of the artists to unite people across different British cultures within the UK was tested under the increasing stress of social division as health and social inequalities widened in the 1980s.

The 1990s would see a New Labour government take power and promote 'social cohesion' through policies of 'inclusion' (Geddes, 2000). Devolution was a policy strand thought to contribute to this wider policy aim since it was intended to "bring government closer to the people," providing a way to "make our politics more inclusive and put power in the hands of the people, where it belongs" (Blair, 1999b). However, class was not a political concept that was deemed useful to this end, with Tony Blair announcing in conclusive terms that "The class war is over" (Blair, 1999a). Rather, the idea of meritocracy was advanced, with equal opportunities promoted through education as citizens were urged to become socially mobile in a new 'stakeholder society' (Blair, 1997).

The first decade under New Labour was marked by years of economic boom (1997–2007). The field of practice known as Arts in Health would gain ministerial support at the highest level of government both in

© The Author(s), under exclusive license to Springer Nature   77
Singapore Pte Ltd. 2023
F. Williams, *When Was Arts in Health?*,
https://doi.org/10.1007/978-981-19-3617-3_4

Westminster and across the devolved administrations in this "golden decade" (a phrase used by Blair to describe the funding of the arts sector across this period).[1] Following the financial crash of 2008, policies of austerity would re-frame this area of practice on a cost effective, even voluntary basis—part of a wider drive to shrink the size of the state through the creation of a so-called "big society" (Cameron, 2010). As the following narratives will reveal, these dynamic renderings of the scale of the state would impact powerfully on how those working across Arts in Health would reconceive their role and purpose.

CLOSURES AND OPENINGS

Two projects became influential exemplars of Arts in Health practice just prior to the election of New Labour in 1997. START is a mental health community arts project, begun in Salford in Greater Manchester in the mid-1980s, held up today "as an international exemplar in this field" (Parkinson, 2011: 22), while another project set-up in a multicultural area of the East End of London, at Bromley-By-Bow, is similarly claimed as "one of the finest examples of an integrated health and community hub".[2] These two projects can be seen as different attempts to address the sense of social and economic malaise concentrated in inner city areas in the 1980s (detailed in the last chapter). This spatialisation took on new significance following the "1981 urban uprisings", historians charting "the privatisation of the struggle" note, since these disturbances "pulled more activists into the local state" (Schofield et al., 2021: 207). Local government became the tier on which political demands for Arts in Health could be advanced and, and in some instances, successfully met.

Originating in the interregnum between Thatcher and Blair, these two projects reveal nuanced responses to the "expressive revolution" of the 1970s and political resistances of the 1980s. They point to the change of government in 1997 as a continuum as much as it marked a decisive break with the past. As Margaret Thatcher would go on to claim, Tony Blair and New Labour were her "greatest achievement" since "we forced our opponents to change their minds".[3] This was an assertion that has been also subsequently acknowledged by Blair. "I always thought my job was to build on some of the things she had done rather than reverse them" (Blair, 2013).[4] Such continuities are discussed in terms of how they represent Labour's turn towards neoliberalism to lesser or greater extent (Panich & Leys, 2001; Wickham-Jones, 2021).

The third sector would play a key role in enabling "historically embedded welfare state provision" to be "discarded in favour of privately capitalised and mixed economy models of cultural and social organisation" (Philips, 2011: 36). Some of this impetus for this came from pressures exerted by social movements, such as the anti-psychiatry movement. The re-configuration of mental healthcare systems within community contexts in the early 1990s, for example, would mark success for those intent on the abolition of the old asylum model. It enabled new types of health organisation to grow in the third sector. Sheltered Training in the Arts (START) was co-founded by Wendy Teal and Langley Brown in 1986, an offshoot of the *Manchester Hospital Arts* group (to which Brown belonged). By 1988, the first ever national centre, *Arts For Health*, was created by Peter Senior through a partnership with Manchester Polytechnic. This new research hub was one where innovative new Arts in Health models, such as START, could find support.

A network of artists' studios in Salford, Oldham and Stockport was developed to cater for patients discharged from Manchester Psychiatric Hospital. Trips to the Peak district were offered to people learning to recover their freedom after release from this institutional setting. Outdoor activities were celebrated through a mosaic at Manchester Royal Infirmary that urged outpatients to *Head for the Hills* (one of many craft skills made available through this organisation, also including textiles, pottery, stained glass and woodwork). Participants in START programmes were referred by healthcare professionals, a fact that has since led to this project being claimed at the first to offer *Arts on Referral* in 1993 (or *Arts on Prescription*, as this working model is now more often called).

Langley Brown was keen to make a break from psychoanalytic therapy models which he saw as pathologising and stigmatising. "We don't call it therapy, we call it art," he insisted. "We are not interested in people's medical history. Illness is a shared negative experience and we offer a shared positive experience through the arts" (Brown, 1993: 5). In a PhD thesis undertaken at Manchester Metropolitan University, he explores this distinction drawing on the work of psychologist David Smail, amongst others. Smail was notable amongst his peers in believing that the scope of any therapeutic treatment needed to be expanded beyond "one's interior world" to acknowledge and "challenge the exterior factors that may have given rise to that distress" (Smail, 1996: 5). He explicitly named Monetarist policy as a cause of social suffering, prompting "questions neither of medicine, nor of 'therapy'. If anything, they can be seen more as questions of morality or, by extension, politics" (Smail, 1996: 6).

Brown assesses START's success relative to the therapeutic 'failure' of mental health services by placing it, as Smail insists we must, within an extended framework of culture, morality and politics:

> Let's remember then that if a mental health service fails, it stands precious little chance of 'rehabilitating' people successfully by drugs and therapy alone; not only are holistic creative and spiritual needs rarely addressed in the circumstances of a discharge from a service, they are singularly ignored in our *culture as a whole* (Brown, 1993: 8 *my italics*)

START was established at a time when many psychiatric hospitals were being closed, a fact acknowledged by Peter Senior as a factor in its (over) subscription. "Projects like START should play an increasingly important part in providing alternative resources" for the "growing number of patients being discharged" (Senior & Croall, 1995: 45). Meeting this need was not without risk, we can note, since some critics had always seen de-institutionalisation as a cover for funding cuts. "An unholy alliance of therapeutic radicals and fiscal conservatives" (Bachrach, 1978: 5). One historic overview is provided by The Kings Fund where a paper observes that while "the closure of the asylum system was a success... the model of community care has undergone a number of changes in light of emerging knowledge and developments in the social context of mental health care provision" (Gilbert & Peck, 2014: 2).

Questions of funding lay at the heart of understanding how social contexts were (mis)perceived to offer 'care in the community', with local authorities taking on the financial responsibility for patients discharged from NHS institutions. The de-institutionalisation of NHS psychiatric hospitals was subsequently proven to have been costly in both human and financial terms. This prompted a reassessment of the need to "place the experience of the service user in the context of wider socio-economic and political change" (Turner et al., 2015: 599). Activists in social movements were rarely able to offer "adequate alternative community or de-institutional provisions", it has been noted (Philo & Parr, 2018: 242). START's limited capacity suggested that only partial success could be won in local contexts if wider structural frames were left unacknowledged or unexamined.

The creation of the Bromley-By-Bow Health Centre (BBBHC) was also informed by a critique of NHS healthcare services, seeking to offer a new community-informed model of healthcare. But unlike START, this working model sought to restructure local services not through devising 'alternate' provision so much as their innovative 'integration'. In 1984, facing falling congregational numbers in the multicultural East End of London, the Rev. Andrew Mawson decided to re-purpose his dilapidated church hall as a welcoming 'shelter' for a range of local community-based activities. These including childcare provision, studio space for artists as well as workshops for those with learning disabilities to learn new skills. Mawson saw an opportunity to buy a plot of derelict land around the church near the proposed site of a new GP clinic, imagining his centre as a bolt-on "extension" of the clinic.

He tells the story of the creation of the BBBHC by way of personal anecdote, one of many "founding myths" that have subsequently grown around it (Froggett & Chamberlayne, 2003: ix). His motivation, he claims, stemmed from his frustration at the attitudes he found amongst local community workers at the nearby Kingsley Hall (situated next door on this site). Though long abandoned by R.D. Laing, it still acted as a community hub. Mawson found here a "strong sense of rights but little of responsibilities" and a model of working that made "a virtue of endless meetings" involving discussion of "abstract theories of equality or race" (Mawson, 2008: 1). "Liberal" approaches had "run amok", he concluded, those "mirrored in the culture of the public sector" (ibid, p. 1).[5] His subsequent championing of a new dynamic figure—that of the "social entrepreneur"—was based on what he presents as a non-ideological position: "realistic practical action on the ground" (Mawson, 2008: 4). This ran counter to others who while "talking endlessly about making poverty history" were "not prepared to do the hard work or embrace the business logic to do anything about it" (ibid, p. 5). His new health centre would stand as a positive example, if implicit reproach, to failing state systems and the Liberal attitudes that he believed underwrote them.

Doctors would work to deliver care while working alongside artists and community activists "under one roof" here (not wholly removed from Laing's idea, albeit an integration struck on very different terms). Heralded today as a "descendent" of *The Peckham Experiment* (Conford, 2020), this "holistic" approach to local community health would be facilitated through a new, bespoke architectural form: "a welcoming environment and quality furnishings, with hard work, enterprise and creativity at its heart, not ideology and theory".[6]

The new centre's design drew on a range of cultural motifs for inspiration, farmyard barn as well as Roman civic forum.[7] It was informed by the cultural trend of post-modernism, with unusual clock tower design, borrowed from medieval examples in the Italian village of San Gimignano. This eclectic ethos made good use of "cultural relativism" in order to circumvent any hostility towards "cultural artefacts that represent state or religious authority"—especially useful, given the multi-faith, ethnically diverse local population in East London. (7) Contemporary theorists, we can note, have since characterised post-modernism as the "Trojan horse" that allowed "a rapacious new kind of capitalism" to borrow cultural vernaculars across time and place, with design features grabbed indeed, from "everywhere" (Jeffries, 2021). The ironic playfulness of Post Modernism, Stuart Jeffries contends, served as seductive trope through which "deregulated markets could be smuggled into public institutions" (ibid, 0) (Fig. 4.1).[8]

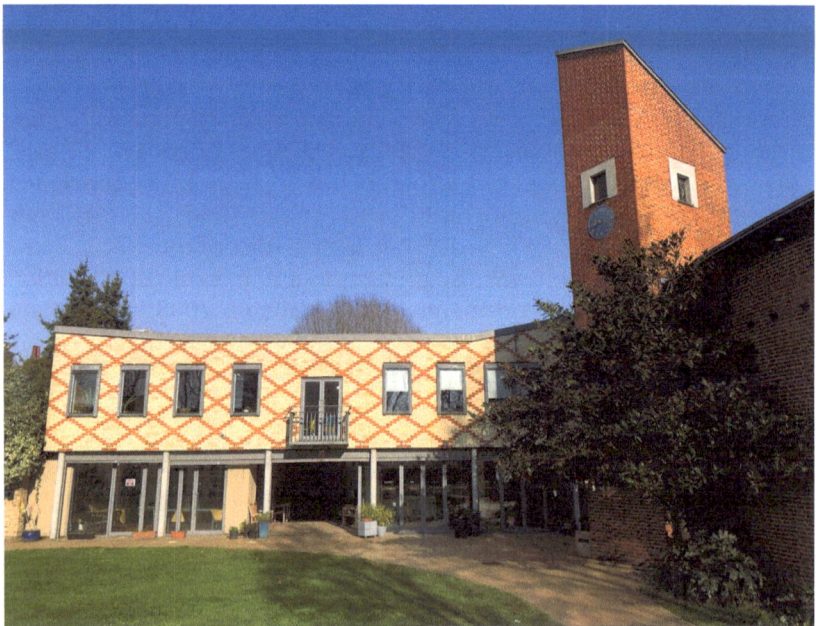

Fig. 4.1   The Bromley-By-Bow Health Centre, with unusual clock tower, fitted around an internal courtyard and external gardens

Public ownership was always raised by Mawson as a potential obstacle to his project's aim—an objection which prompted one Health Minister to ask upon visiting the site in 2003, "Where is the NHS sign?" (9)[9] Mawson suggested that the BBBHC be owned as a trust, an idea dismissed by the local health authority on the basis that it was "not equitable" to allow "one group of individuals to take healthcare provision into their own hands" (Conford, 2020: 425). It was only at the behest and direct intervention of the then Conservative Health Minister (Brian Mawhinny) that funding for doctors was provided over three years by the local authority. The new building opened its doors to local people in 1997 and was quickly championed by the incoming New Labour government as the prototype for hundreds of other *Health Living Centres* across the whole of the UK.[10]

New Labour's enthusiasm for this project was part of their desire to "modernize" the NHS, one that acknowledged the role of third sector agencies in supporting public health. A fresh report, *Inequalities in Health* (1997), authored by Donald Acheson, pointed to social class as a social determinant of health (much as The Black Report had done, a decade earlier). "Although the last 20 years have brought a marked increase in prosperity and substantial reductions in mortality to the people of the country as a whole, the gap in health between those at the top and bottom of the social scale has widened" (Acheson, 1997). This time around, the findings of this report found a more receptive ministerial audience and informed a new policy approach undertaken by the Department of Health (Our Healthier Nation, 1999). An explicit recognition of the role of culture in promoting public health appeared in an NHS Health Education Authority report published in 2000. This concluded that:

> The solutions to major public health problems… will require interventions which cut across sectors to take account of the broader social, cultural, economic, political and physical environments which shape people's experiences of health and wellbeing (Art for Health, 2000)

The election of New Labour allowed BBBHC to exemplify a joint private-public finance approach, one which saw Mawson promote "enterprise as a tool for economic development in deprived communities," congruent with Blair's advancement of a *Third Way*.

A Declaration of Intent

The election of Tony Blair as Prime Minister offered opportunity for others, beyond Andrew Mawson, intent on establishing a place for the arts and culture within health and education systems at this time. The millennium is commonly located as a "turning point" for the field of Arts in Health, (Clift et al., 2009: 9), a period when regional groupings agreed to pursue shared national agenda. Two so-called 'Windsor Conferences' (in 1998 and 1999) saw the fortunes of those working in the humanities in healthcare forge links with the new *esprit du jour* represented by the New Labour government.[11] *The Windsor Declaration for the Humanities in Healthcare* enthusiastically proposed that "elevating the arts, health and wellbeing into a pivotal role across the spectrum of health care may be the real third way for health" (Philipp et al., 1999: 6). The opportunity provided by the 'third way' was, however, complicated by new tiers of government across the 'four nations'.

The years leading up the millennium had seen referendums staged to offer more political autonomy to those living in these parts of the UK, those most negatively impacted by Thatcher's economic and industrial policies. Acts of Devolution passed through Parliament and gave new powers to legislative bodies based in Wales, Scotland and Northern Ireland. Both 'Arts' and 'Health' fell under these devolved jurisdictions, with opportunity presented for policy latitude in how Arts in Health could be enacted across tiers of government (now subject to alternate, if parallel, structures of democratic accountability). These constitutional developments brought the discourse of Arts in Health into a more tangled relationship with variegated and more complex forms of political power.

Nothing encapsulates this complexity better, perhaps, than the basis on which a new 'national' network for Arts in Health practitioners was formed. Prime amongst the recommendations made by *The Windsor Declaration* was the need for such a body. The National Network for Arts in Health (NNAH) was established in the millennial year of 2000. According to its first director, this was the moment when "a unified voice enabling collective action" was made possible for the first time (Dose, 2006: 110). Up until this point, only "disparate individuals" had operated "in a vacuum" with no government support (ibid, p. 110). But no distinction was made then—or has been since—to explain why the NNAH was only ever conceived as an English body and not a British one. Neither was NNAH, strictly speaking, the first 'national' body for Arts in Health since

Manchester's *Arts For Health* had been set up on a UK-wide basis 12 years earlier.

No mention of devolution is made in *The Windsor Declaration*.[12] It does, however, give a detailed account of how its own constitutional arrangement was arrived at. A meeting between two powerful men is credited here as a catalyst for action bringing Arts and Health together through enlisting the support of successive government ministers. The UK's Chief Medical Officer (Kenneth Calman) met the Conservative Minister for Health (Gerry Malone) in 1996 to discuss the "increasing interest" in "arts in healthcare". Together they agreed to set up of a steering group that could find ways to "take forward the new therapeutic approach" (Philipp et al., 1998: 9). This working group comprised Dr Robin Philipp and Professor Michael Baum (both eminent physicians) alongside Rev. Andrew Mawson (founder of the BBBHC) and Professor John Wyn Owen, Secretary of the Nuffield Trust, (who agreed financial support for the Windsor conferences through this role).

Following the change in government in 1997, the impetus for arts in healthcare did not stall but continued apace. The drive towards embedding Arts in Health through government policy appeared to transcend party political difference. Indeed, Mawson's health centre was described as "a bridgehead between New Conservatism and New Labour" (Chamberlayne & Rupp, 2007: 1). The NNAH was conceived as a "federal arrangement" of equal regional bodies based within England not an alliance of devolved national bodies working together on an equal basis. There was uncertainly whether "individuals should relate to the umbrella organisation via a federation of centres that reflect their geographical location or their special interests" (ibid, 53). In the end, the steering group borrowed a model from UNESCO in order to propose that "the national body should have a federal structure consisting of partner centres with one of these acting as a national co-ordinating centre" (Philipps et al., 1998: 54). Durham University was chosen as the site for a new *Centre for Arts and Humanities in Health and Medicine* in 2001, with Mike White appointed as its first director.

Little attention is given in *The Windsor Declaration* to the way that inequality informs national or place-based contexts or population health, despite one contributor noting how "national barriers lose their importance as trade and investment, communication and cultures cross boundaries" (Philipp et al., 1998: 7). Such omissions are even more notable in retrospect given that the differences in mortality rates across areas of the

UK had first led researchers to label the study of health inequality by way of place. Research undertaken into population health in the late 1980s could find no explanation for the high mortality levels found in Glasgow relative to other UK cities with similar socioeconomic profiles—a mystery dubbed the Glasgow, or 'Scottish effect'.[13]

Though left un-addressed through its own institutional formation, the field of Arts in Health was increasingly underpinned by epidemiological research into health and mortality 'gaps' across different populations living in different geographic regions. Inequality was identified as an 'affliction' besetting 'unhealthy societies' (Wilkinson, 1996). Research into health inequality was used to underpin a range of UK government policies—including the creation of Health Action Zones (HAZs) in poorer areas as well as the creation of hundreds of new Healthy Living Centres across the country. Funded by the new National Lottery and based squarely on the BBBHC model, Healthy Living Centres were financially supported for three years. Few, however, went on to become self-sustainable after this initial period of government funding.[14]

While evidence of the problem of health inequality was becoming clearer through epidemiological research, effective political solutions proved much harder to implement. The failure of the national roll-out of the Healthy Living Centre programme suggests that BBBHC may have better been regarded as a unique local case study rather than a prototype suitable to be 'scaled-up' at national level. Mawson put the policy failure down to "confused ideas and lack of leadership", while public health researchers identified "unrealistic expectations" (Judge & Bauld, 2006). The latter urged that "greater efforts be made to learn from expensive policy failure such as this and that future initiatives" be based on better evidence (ibid, 341).

THE STUFF OF DREAMS

Funding issues, relative to election cycles, increasingly lay at the heart of the strategic choices chosen by those working to promote the field of Arts in Health. One suggestion floated not long after the millennial moment offered new hope. A Lancet editorial quoted Ivan Illich's ideas of 'adaptation' to make the budgetary case for Arts in Health in 2002. A mere 0.5 per cent transfer from the NHS budget to Arts Council England would hold transformative potential, Richard Smith argued. "If health is about adaptation… then the arts may be more potent than anything medicine has to offer" (Smith, 2002: 1432). This simple diversion would have increased Arts Council England's budget by 70 per cent, signalling a profound change in thinking and adaptation—a prospect heralded by Mike White as "the stuff of dreams" (White, 2009: 4).

Though this redirection of resource never came to pass, ten years of hard lobbying appeared to yield a significant prize when Peter Hewitt, then Executive Director of Arts Council England (ACE), published a *Prospectus for Arts in Health in* 2008. This was a document signed by both junior ministers in the Departments for Culture, Media and Sport (DCMS) and Department of Health. It marked the first formal co-joining of the arts and health sectors at this ministerial level through a shared policy document. The Prospectus rejected the idea of Arts in Health as "fringe activity", instead welcoming creative activities into the centre of the Department of Health's remit. This assertion was evidenced by "hundreds of research projects, organisations and individuals" that pointed to how the arts might form "an integral part of the *nature and quality* of the services we provide" (ibid, p. *my italics*). These included projects made possible "through prescription", with artists credited as having "a profound impact on people's health" not only "in hospitals and health centres," but within "GP practices and across the community" too (2006, p. 10).

Though less well-documented, similar processes of the assimilation of Arts in Health projects into devolved government policy were also underway in Scotland, Wales and Northern Ireland—all of whom developed their own Arts in Health programmes and bodies.[15] A conference hosted by Arts Council Wales (ACW) in 2006 kick-started a steering group to develop a joint strategy for Arts and Health with The Welsh Assembly. This led to the adoption of an *Action Plan for Wales*, supported by both Health and Culture ministers in the Welsh Government at this time (ACW, 2009).[16] Wales' adopted policy approach replicated, rather than radically diverged, from Westminster's during these years in relation to the Arts in Health agenda.

From this auspicious moment, many setbacks commenced. Most significant amongst these was the global economic crisis of 2008, but also the earlier financial collapse in 2006 of NNAH. This was an organisational bankruptcy that took place despite NNAH being run for less than the salary of a single NHS General Practitioner it was painfully observed, with 'lessons' needing to be learned (Dose, 2006). The broader financial crash prompted a revised approach to public spending, marking a 'culture crash' for creative practitioners across the globe (Timberg, 2015). Fears were articulated around the impact of the financial crisis on artist's sense of autonomy. "If working in culture becomes something only for the wealthy or those supported by corporate patronage," one US author on this topic warned in response at this time, "we lose the independent perspective that artistry is based on" (ibid, p. 14).

In an academic paper jointly authored by leading actors in the field in 2008, questions were asked about the "state of arts in health" at this uncertain moment (Clift et al., 2009). Dialogues begin to emerge around to what extent Arts in Health could act as a genuine "agent of social transformation or a mere instrumental tool" of government (White, 2009: 14). The authors felt a particular need to rebut the arguments of one critic who directly attacked Arts in Health as a "misleading amalgamation" of "activities and effects" (Mirza, 2006: 63).

CULTURE VULTURES

Published by a Right of centre think tank (*The Policy Exchange*), Munira Mirza edited a collection of essays titled *Culture Vultures: Is UK Arts Policy Damaging the Arts?* (2006). She questioned the field's close relationship to governmental power and accused the Arts in Health lobby of adopting a (hidden) political agenda. She also questioned the fundamental claim that community art helps "empower local people" (2006: 65). In an echo of Michael Heseltine's phrasing, *It Took a Riot*, she references rioting to parody community arts' radical intention and the role of the state in supporting it:

> If art is truly doing its job, might we not also see more rioting in the streets and social unrest? Of course, this possibility does not even enter into the discussion, because the implication for arts and health projects is clear: they are not about using the arts to express a greater truth about ourselves, but to manage our emotional lives and even, perhaps, to placate us (Mirza, 2006: 105)

Complaints of uncritical collusion with governmental agendas became more frequent from this point onwards in England, if not in Wales (which remained the 'land of the pulled punch' due to the election of back-to-back Labour administrations).[17] Criticism began to also emerge from within the field in England, not only actors on The New Right. Mike White also asked, for example, if New Labour's audit culture was negatively impacting on Arts and Health practice. He complained of Hospital Care Trusts being "so target driven" that the vitality of art practice was being placed at risk through New Managerialism (White, 2006: 50). Arts in Health projects were becoming so instrumentalised that there was little "breathing space" to "explore what makes for effective public engagement of creativity with health" he asserted (ibid, 51). White extended Langley Brown's notion of pathology beyond the clinic to name what he called the "pathology of the environment" (White, 2011). He quotes epidemiologist Michael Marmot on this point, whose influential report *Fair Society Healthy Lives* was published in 2010. Marmot insisted that social determinants of health be acted upon to address health inequalities. A priority of future health policy, White said, should be to "create and develop healthy and sustainable places and communities," noting pointedly that the determinants of health are "affected by the socio-political and cultural context in which they sit" (White, 2011: 45).

Issues of scale, as well as socio-political context, are also raised as potentially problematic at this time. The degree to which Arts in Health activities could be considered "substantial" when set alongside mainstream healthcare provision was questioned (Clift et al., 2009: 9). This would prove the first of many comparisons increasingly made around comparative value for money between the culture and health sectors. Fears were raised that as cuts in public expenditure took effect, the field would lay itself vulnerable to accusations that arts activities were a frivolous luxury compared to 'frontline' health services considered more essential.

The press coverage of one artwork commissioned to sit outside a London hospital threatened the positive public reputation the field had built for itself. A marble sculpture by artist John Aiken was purchased by one NHS Trust for £70,000 in 2005, notoriously nicknamed 'the gallstone' by one tabloid newspaper. Such coverage illustrated how the proposal of Arts in Health as unaffordable luxury was one with potential to foster public hostility. "Arts in health is not about replacing a dialyser with a Dalí" one defender took up the comparison in defence of Paintings in Hospitals (Walshaw, 2017). A new resolve, at any rate, to win funding developed out of the demise of the NNAH, a determination forged within a challenging new economic climate of fiscal constraint (Fig. 4.2).

New ways of thinking about 'social art practice' were emerging at this time. These rejected longer traditions of object-making but for different reasons to those advanced in the tabloid press. "Parting from the traditions of object-making," artists adopted "a performative, process-based approach" acting "as 'context providers' rather than 'content providers'," one US critic proposed (Kester, 2004: 153). This new 'dialogic' and 'littoral' art placed emphasis on art's discursive, performative and pedagogic potentials.

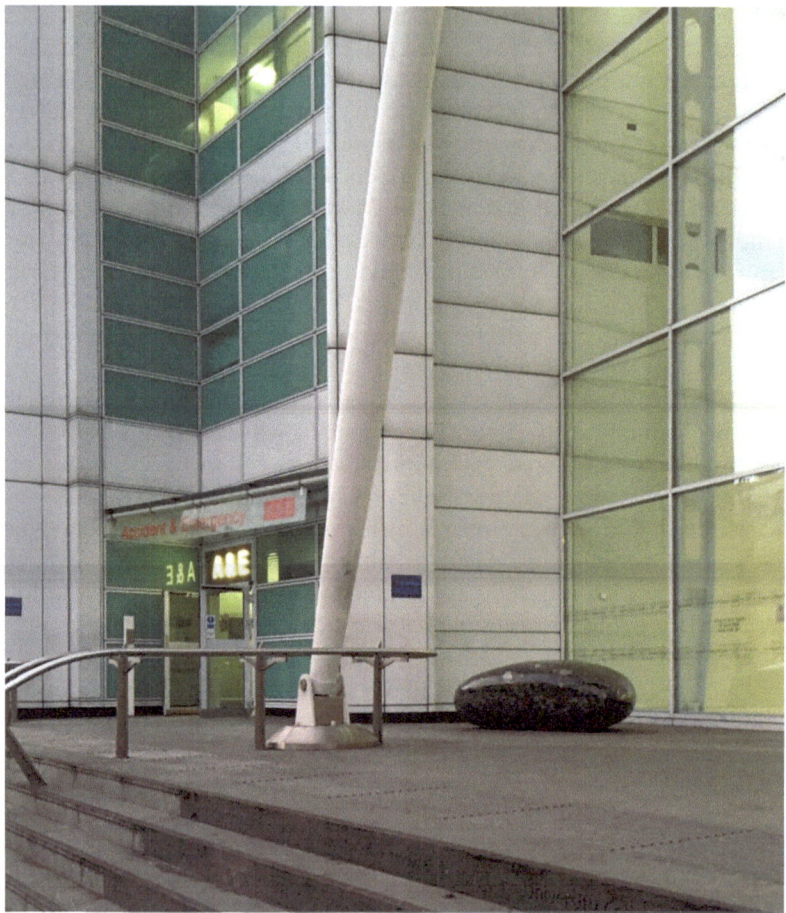

Fig. 4.2   'The gallstone' installed at University College Hospital in 2005

Theories around 'socially engaged' art practice as the vehicle for social change were championed alongside New Labour's cultural policy which also placed an emphasis on 'Education, Education, Education' (Blair, 2001). In 2005, the New Labour government announced a £9.4 million investment in museum and gallery education programmes. Researcher

Francois Matarasso forged direct links between government policy and participatory art through his research, holding faith in the transformative power of what he would go on to call, a "restless art" (Matarasso, 2019). The "normalisation of participatory art" through government policy was a "battle" that had been "won", he affirmed in 2019. It represents "a remarkable achievement" that has led to "millions of lives" being "changed for the better in small ways and large" (ibid, p. 25).

Many others working in the early 2000s felt the need to make a clear distinction between artistic and social aims detecting "a worrying co-opting of museums and galleries by a New Labour political culture in the service of distinctly New Labour ends" (Morton, 2006). Curators such as Miwon Kwon had long drawn a line between what she called the "bureaucratic" agency enabled via "prescribed" social art projects, as opposed to those art practices which sought to throw the idea of community into question (Kwon, 2002). Only approaches allowing participants the opportunity for "critical epiphany" could "produce non-essentialist subjects", Grant Kester similarly argued (Kester, 2004: 154). Artists could promote the:

> capacity of tightly knit communities to approach difference from a position of dialogical openness rather than defensive hostility, forming provisional alliances across boundaries of race, ethnicity and geography. (ibid)

Making related points to those made by art critics above, social scientists similarly argued that "building community has become a fetishist issue for all tiers of government" (Clements et al., 2008: 4). "The way the debate is framed has nothing to do with real community development but concerns social engineering" (ibid, 4). These authors perceived a controlling state, one whose agents deploy a "managerial approach to community development", one that "short-circuits" social and political realities (5). Art critic Paulo Merli objected to the moral high tone adopted by "new missionaries", towards the poor, making a distinction between the "original phenomena of community arts"—seen to be part of an authentic, "spontaneous movement" as opposed to the state's "revival" of this idea as part of a governmental push for "cultural participation" (Merli, 2002: 4).

The adoption of policies of participation struck on these terms prompted some art curators to respond to community need by way of semi-illicit strategies. The subversive notion of the 'para-site', drew on feminist critiques of the gallery which pointed to the adoption of covert strategies within unjust institutional infrastructures (Allen, 2008) as well as art traditions of institutional critique. Janna Graham used her position within the organisational hierarchy of The Serpentine Gallery to support local diaspora communities through the creation of *The Centre for Possible Studies*. Sited in one of London's Royal Parks' in West London, she forged strong links with those living 'On the Edgware Road' many of whom were connected, through their communities, to the Arab Uprisings in Egypt unfolding at this time. Graham saw opportunity to: "open up of political dynamics in the local" through "a series of global comings and goings and... subversive diplomacies".[18]

Graham rejected the "dominant narrative" whereby the community arts movement was "relegated to the realm of the naïve... incorporated into hegemonic culture" (Graham, 2014: 1). Rather, she kept open the possibility that resources could be smuggled from the "silos of high culture" to support "local and minority experience", albeit via skewed infrastructures (ibid, p. 2). Speaking of the contradiction of (her own) institutional role, she situated herself amongst others who "align themselves with social justice movements" and who work "in collaboration with working-class communities" but who "schizophrenically find themselves para-siting the realms of corporate and cultural elites" (ibid, p. 3). She notes the Janus face of the contemporary art gallery as one keen to "showcase socially progressive art" but which is nevertheless orientated, through its funding structures, towards:

> securing social hierarchy by providing greater levels of access and influence to corporations, real estate developers, wealthy individuals, and paternalistic state policies. (ibid, p. 3)

Graham developed one influential Arts in Health project whose scope was both pedagogic and dialogic. *Art+Care: A Future* (2013) went "beyond providing a service for the care sector," to "argue that art has a role to play in challenging the marginalisation of the aged". It simultaneously aimed to "provoke fundamental questions in the field of art" (ibid, p. 5). Greater awareness, amongst project stakeholders, of the structural conditions in which they jointly operated was actively fostered through this discursive project—one which was able to hold and explore conflicting social and financial needs. This project—and others like it—insisted on interpretative frameworks being kept open for what might constitute any exchange of knowledge between arts-health bodies. They rejected any single treatment model as indicator of social value, arguing for productive and healthy agonism—those borne of "creative collisions" (Rooke, 2011).

This insistence on the value of conflict and critique was made in the face of calls, by some within the Arts in Health field, that 'gold standard' research methods be brought to bear upon the efficacy of (art) interventions in order to better secure both their legitimacy and funding (Clift et al., 2009; Fancourt, 2017). This emphasised the benefit of deploying narrower biomedical metrics to measure impact as these were regarded as practical and realistic since "attempting to change that would require a seismic shift" (Fancourt, 2017: 200). Some queried the basis on which scientific methods could be held as 'trustworthy' (Ravetz &Gregory, 2018). While others repeated long-standing doubts as to whether generating 'a 'wealth of evidence' would serve to distract from the need to 'question targets' and query high expectations (Hope, 2011: 31).

Early, dedicated Arts in Health organisations, such as START, began to become exceptions to the rule in upholding 'health' as their core objective—regardless of how it was measured or assessed. Rather, Arts in Health projects increasingly occupied gallery and museum contexts, often by way of the side-doors marked 'Education' or 'Outreach'. Situated in these 'demimonde' secondary spaces (Kester, 2012), Arts in Health was implicated in subtle infighting embodied by 'The New Institution' (Farquharson, 2006; Raunig, 2009). Curatorial deliberations were held to provide the means by which orthodox gallery hierarchies could be scrambled: "expressed both spatially and temporally in terms of how institutions' hardware (their buildings) and software (their schedules) are apportioned" (Farqurson, 2006: 5). For one enthusiastic proponent, such fluid programming could "side step" the inherent problematics of the gallery since:

> If white-walled rooms are the site for exhibitions one week, a recording studio or political workshop the next, then it is no longer the container that defines the contents as art, but the contents that determine the identity of the container. (ibid, p. x)

Indeed, Alex Farquarson found resonance in his approach with "the anti-psychiatry movement of the 1960s and the associated work of R. D. Laing and Felix Guttari" (ibid, 2). But for others, the un-demarcated zones of The New Institution continued to replicate processes of marginalisation, simply presenting them in more camouflaged form (Moersch, 2011). Using a memorable phrase, gallery educator Carmen Moersch identified the 'new' curatorial interest in education and health by way of a metaphor of colonialism, comparing it to how "Columbus 'discovered' America"—a novelty better seen as the result of the art world's "endless demand for the circulation of 'the new' than any deep or respectful engagement" (ibid, p. 2).

Regardless of conclusions drawn from these debates—strung between art theory, cultural policy and public health discourses—the struggle to make the gallery space fit for (social) purpose show how Arts in Health grew on certain terms, for certain reasons, by way of certain institutional structures. Opportunism was a motivation that always presented itself for arts organisations in their adoption of the 'health agenda' since "austerity means that arts organisations… facing significant cuts, look to see new trends that may inform project delivery" (Rooke, 2011: 2).

A scholarly retrospective view is offered by Professor Alan Bleakley, writing about the influence of The Windsor Declaration in a book devoted to *Medicine Health and the Arts* (Bleakley, 2014). He charts how various strands of practice—those that fell under the "umbrella" term of Arts in Health—could not cohere and hold. Distinct new categories and subfields came about as the result of "fault lines" reflective of diverse needs; pedagogic, clinical, creative and academic. These conflicts led to a "divergence" of interests and splits into separate fields and strands. While arts curricula were successfully embedded in medical education, it has led to a "nuanced" rather than a "fundamental critique" of the medical knowledge, Bleakley ruefully observes (2014: 23).

DEEPER CUTS

While the millennium was thought auspicious for the field of Arts in Health, the year of 2011 was seen more darkly as ushering in perils and threats—indeed, a time when it "seemed like the national arts and health agenda might have already run out of steam" (Parkinson & White, 2013). A general election in 2011 saw a new coalition government elected comprising Conservatives and Liberal Democrats. As in 1997, this change of administration brought policies different to those preceding it, but many that were consistent and continuous. The foundations of Cameron's 'Big Society' were already "being laid in the final term of the Labour government" (White & Robson, 2011).

One continuity was represented by David Cameron's adoption of behavioural economics in the area of public health. His championing of 'nudge theory' led him to establish a bespoke policy unit designed to change the way citizens make healthy choices. This approach posited the exercise of free choice within the frameworks of "choice architectures" (Thaler et al., 2010). Financial incentives were a key element in this approach, one fully supported by the (then) Chancellor, George Osborne. *The Nudge Unit* was created in the same year as the introduction of a new auditing tool, *The National Well-being Index*.

This novel body was set up to gather annual statistics, using the subjective measurement of 'well-being' set alongside those of economic growth. Its introduction drew on arguments which questioned gross domestic product (GDP) as the primary indicator of government policy success (Laylard, 2011). David Cameron took on this idea and used it as part of his mission to repurpose The Conservative Party as a force for progressive change (keen to relinquish its former reputation as 'the nasty party' of the 1980s). This strategy involved him acknowledging limits to the power of the market in relation to health, championing the 'quality of culture':

> Wellbeing can't be measured by money or traded in markets. It's about the beauty of our surroundings, the quality of our culture and, above all, the strength of our relationships. (Cameron, 2010)

Together these joint initiatives marked important policy shifts for those Arts in Health. They complimented Cameron's main policy plank of a 'big society' whereby it was affirmed that "only when people and communities are given more power and take more responsibility can we achieve fairness" (Cameron, 2010). A "radical devolution of power" was identified as a way of delivering this vision (Cameron, 2010: 6) with the goal of 'well-being' and process of 'devolution' linked at the beginning of a decade which would see deeper cuts to local authority spending.

A re-configured national network, *The National Alliance for Arts, Health and Wellbeing* (NAAHW), was created in 2012, offering a new definition of Arts in Health incorporated the word 'well-being' into its title. The London Arts in Health Forum (LAHF) led the drive to bring together this new English network, amongst whom internal divisions now began to be felt and publicly expressed. The *Charter for Arts, Health and Well-being* produced by the LAHF situated the field in the current political and economic "climate", which it claimed "forced a reassessment of human priorities" (Jackson, 2012). As "well-being is a declared government priority," the Charter stated, Arts in Health can "offer a professional, value-for-money contribution to mainstream health care" (Jackson, 2012: 2).

Northern English perspectives gave rise to a different view and rationale. Produced in the same year by The North West Arts and Health Network, alternate *Arts and Health Manifestos* were published, edited by Clive Parkinson, through Manchester Metropolitan University. While this supported the premise that the arts contribute positively to health, the manifesto emphatically contradicts The Charter in other respects. "It is not about reducing the arts to a cost-effective solution" (Parkinson, 2011, 2012). These texts suggested that Arts in Health work towards "a better, not a bigger, society". The difference of emphasis between those groups based in the North and South of England was perhaps not so coincidental given that Northern regions were disproportionately affected by the policies of austerity, implemented by way of Labour councils based in some of the poorest areas. Mike White characterised this moment in time as one which presented "a fork in the road" for those working Arts in Health (White, 2014). He openly challenged the field's "mis-direction" in an article which reflected on the role of this field of practice in a "new landscape". While one road followed The Lantern Way (of continued community arts development), the other, he cautioned, would lead to:

> probable damnation by way of *austerity culture*, a narrowing definition of accredited practice, and evidence calls that are signalled through a medical model of health. (White, 2014: 1 *my italics*)

As the deleterious social and health impacts of policies of austerity began to be felt, Mike White saw little cause for optimism in the transfer for responsibility for public health from national, to local government as this would likely "demonstrate even more the development of health service delivery by hybrid professions and partnerships" (White, 2014: 3).

His doubts were shared by some public health researchers writing at this time who also identified a "failure to question the balance of power between public services, communities and corporate interests" (Friedli, 2012: 10). In focusing on the failures of the state, the destructive impacts of "free market capitalism" were left "off the hook", exposing some regions to the "abandonment of both the market and the state" (Friedli, 2012: 8). Local services provided by the NHS were also, at this time, being made subject to 'reforms' by way of Andrew Lansley's internal NHS restructuring made through *Health and Social Care Act (2012)*. This extended competition within the 'internal market' of the NHS with GP consortia taking on the management of local healthcare budgets.[19] New Clinical Commissioning Groups (CCGs) dictated the contractual terms on which local services—including those that might deploy arts for health approaches—were bought, valued and proven to 'work'.

Two years on from the passing of Lansley's controversial piece of legislation (which was rejected in Wales by the devolved government), local government in England was also offered the opportunity, for the first time since the 1930s, to gain control of the NHS and social care budgets at local authority level. The policy of regional devolution was pioneered by the architect of austerity, George Osborne. He struck the first secret 'devo deal' with Greater Manchester city leaders in 2015 with no recourse to any referenda or democratic vote. Labour city leaders believed they could meet the bottom line though service innovation, gaining more power and autonomy for themselves in the process. 'Devo-Manc' was a play on words intended to echo the promise of 'Devo-Max'—the wider powers promised to the Scottish government to face down the threat posed by the independence vote of 2014.[20] While purportedly offering greater autonomy for the city region, this new form of English devolution placed new fiscal responsibilities onto those working to secure better health in Greater Manchester—a *fait accompli* that allowed for no rejection of austerity, rather its accommodation as impetus for arts-health innovation.

Mike White and Clive Parkinson continued to underline health inequality as the focus through which participatory arts might promote public health, expanding their proposal beyond the UK. They chided those whose "internal focus" was trained solely on "funding problems" at the expense of exploring "cross national collaboration" with others beyond the English-speaking world (Parkinson & White, 2013). Other actors, meanwhile, advanced the Arts in Health agenda more in line with the new Coalition government and its political ethos. "We've already linked the arts with health economics, a vital step to establish cost effectiveness, and we've developed a planning tool and a standards of evidence framework" (Joss, 2014).

Tim Joss held a distaste for state subsidy, casting it a "dependency" that could "skew" the market, "for no good reason" (Joss, 2008: 85). Rather, he championed commercial and "popular" art forms as offering better opportunity for "closer engagement", especially with "multicultural" publics in the UK (ibid, 8). In a text of 2008 titled *New Flow*, Joss sets out his approach. He revisits the early history of the Arts Council of Great Britain to chime with commentators on The Left: "arts councils have great difficulty with popular culture" (ibid, 84).[21] He further upholds criticism of The Arts sector as "elitist" in order to insist on dismantling the current system of state support. Reviving the idea of Third Way with renewed enthusiasm, Joss presents these (neoliberal) policies as those best embraced since they are "irreversible".

> The commercial and voluntary sectors are converging and this is now irreversible. National and local government increasingly looks to the voluntary

sector for the delivery of public services. As the boundaries blur, entrepre-
neurial skills will become more important. (Joss, 2008: 8)

Joss was commissioned by Public Health England to develop an evaluation
framework for Arts in Health in 2015, an initiative supplemented by an
online 'tool' developed by his own company (Aesop). The so-named *Aesop
marketplace* provided a virtual "dating" site for Health commissioners to
access artist-led projects on a speculative, service provision basis. At an
event for these combined initiatives, the Secretary of State for Health
(Jeremy Hunt) spoke alongside Arts Council England's Chief Executive
(Peter Bazelgette) to affirm Arts in Health on the terms set out by Joss,
namely "cost effective... evidence-based... capable of going to scale" (Joss,
2016). (There are precepts, we can one, that were similarly advanced by
Arts Council Wales whose mapping report of Arts in Health in Wales of
2017 further echoes these aims.) Hunt collated two worthy aspirations as
one, praising Arts in Health programmes on the basis that they not only
presented better alternates to pills, but were "cheaper than drugs". This
affirmation was made to the deep unease of those keen to ensure artist's
financial remuneration reflect the value of their contribution to this field
of work.

   In the same year, the NHS was radically re-framed by its Chief Executive,
Simon Stephens. The *Five Year Forward Plan* (2014) for the NHS suggested that the NHS should be seen a "as a social movement", one that
might enable "a shift in power to patients and citizens" (NHS, 2014: 14).
Three million pounds was allocated to three think tanks to encourage
patients and health workers alike to adopt and understand social movement theory and strategies.[22] Despite being initiated and fully funded by
the NHS, a report produced by NETSA (Del Castillo et al., 2016) asserted,
without any irony, that social movements:

> bubble up outside of formal institutions and from beyond established power
> structures. They challenge and disrupt. They are restless and determined.
> They often make society, elites and institutions deeply uncomfortable as
> they challenge accepted values, priorities and procedures. (Del Castello &
> Kahn, 2016: 5)

CODA: CREATIVE HEALTH

This, then, was the challenging political and economic context in which
the APPGAHW report began to be researched in 2014, presented to a
new government in a time of deepening political crisis. The Brexit

referendum result of 2016 saw David Cameron resign as Prime Minister. With this choice to exit the EU, the future jurisdictions of all UK legislative frameworks were thrown into doubt, particularly those of the devolved nations. These now came under fresh scrutiny by central government, made subject to more 'muscular' iterations of unionism.

The referendum result served to vindicate the belief, long held by key researchers into inequality, that trust had been eroded by ever-widening social inequality in the UK. The result held unwelcome consequence for those in the arts keen to retain an international audience and context for their work, if not necessarily secure arts value within the framework of the international art market. Some warned against a new parochialism taking hold as a result: "There is no point in focusing solely on the local—a suggestion which some in the museum world might pander to in order to heal the Brexit divide" (Gould, 2018). Others argued that Brexit was a political choice only made possible *as a result* of widening economic inequality. Longstanding researchers into inequality, on studying the demographics of the 'Leave' vote, propose that the result should be seen as the symptom of social inequality, one best understood as

> a visceral reaction from those who have felt increasingly powerless as a result of globalisation, widening economic inequalities and a failure of successive UK government administrations to redistribute income and wealth more equitably for more than thirty, almost forty years. (Dorling et al., 2016)

In conclusion then, the twists and turns of the narrative detailed above give a sense of the broad currents on which the category of Arts in Health was created, unified and carried forward, by the institutions and networks through which it has found expression over 20 years (1997–2017). Within this narrative, moments of fracture, risk and dissolution can also be discerned.

Some of the guiding metaphors adopted in the APPGAHW report reveal the field's latest position as a defensive one. Rather than represent the arts as 'social tonic' (White, 2008), the metaphor used to describe the beneficial effect of the arts on our health was an "essential vaccine" (ibid, 30). Using this biomedical term, the APPGAHW report acknowledges the arts as unable to address the structural causes of inequality in the UK:

Arts engagement may be envisaged as a factor that can *mitigate* the effects of health inequalities while policies are implemented to eradicate their causes. (APPGAHW, 2017: 10 *my emphasis*)

Some of the ambivalence of this contingent position is captured by illustrations commissioned for the short report devised by the artist David Shrigley. They speak of a bleaker truth behind the affirmation that "the arts can reconstruct you", namely that the healing of social division within the UK, is *not so* easy since deep cuts and various 'hollowing-outs' have been executed. The social harm of inequality, deepened by a decade of austerity—left unresolved by devolution—shows no sign of being halted, let alone reversed (Fig. 4.3).

In an echo of the motif used to encourage protest in Paris in 1968, one drawing presents a dismembered body as broken shell. But neither bourgeois medicine nor bourgeois art find a mention in the accompanying slogan. (Shrigley is an artist whose work commands high sums.) His images

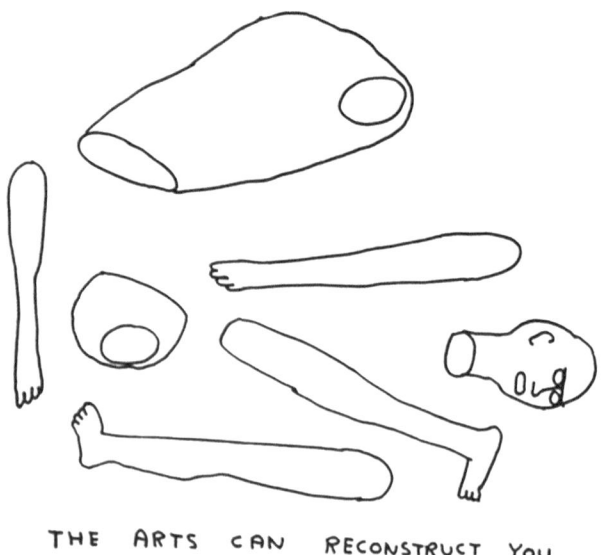

THE ARTS CAN RECONSTRUCT YOU

Fig. 4.3   David Shrigley's illustration for the creative health short report, 2017

belong as much to the international art market as any social movement for health—albeit using a similar vernacular to cartoons drawn by patients to articulate their dis-alienation within the asylum. As such, it represents a fitting illustration for a field of art practice which, though committed to addressing social and health inequality through culture, also adopts the values set by global systems of capital that serve to reproduce and deepen it.

NOTES

1. https://www.theguardian.com/politics/2007/mar/07/uk.artsfunding.
2. According to their own website, it can be noted. https://www.bbbc.org.uk.
3. Conor Burns recounts this response to a question he asked her at a 2002 dinner. https://conservativehome.blogs.com/centreright/2008/04/making-history.html.
4. Blair spoke to the press in tribute to Thatcher in the year of her death: https://www.bbc.co.uk/news/av/uk-politics-22073434.
5. Foundational stories are expanded upon in his book, titled *The Social Entrepreneur: Making Communities Work*, published in 2008.
6. He wrote a short account in an article in the guardian published in 2008. https://www.theguardian.com/society/2008/jan/09/socialenterprises. regeneration.
7. This strategic use of design and these words are those of the architect of the Centre, Gordon MacLaren, quoted by Kip Jones in a case study devoted to the architecture of BBBHC (Jones, 2003: 14).

   McLaren has also gone on to make critical comments about new healthcare architectures becoming too much like "the hospitality sector" in a talk hosted by BBBHC in January 2022. https://www.youtube.com/watch?v=fhMAmrWqexA.
8. Stuart Jeffries broadly argues that postmodernism has resulted in the impossibility of conceiving politics as a communal activity. https://www.thenation.com/article/culture/postmodern-stuart-jeffries.
9. John Reid, visiting in 2003 in his capacity as Health Minister in Tony Blair's government from 2003 to 2005. As recounted by Sam Everington. See: https://www.bmj.com/content/333/7580/gp218.
10. HLCs were funded by the new National Lottery. See Blair's speech on 'healthy living' here: https://www.theguardian.com/society/2006/jul/26/health.politics.
11. So called because they took place in the town of Windsor, near London, funded by the Nuffield Trust.
12. This may be explained by the fact that, as one constitutional historian puts the point, the English 'do not think of themselves as living in a region…'

since England is assumed to be 'the naturally dominant nation' (Bogdanor, 2014).

13. Phrases subsequently abandoned on the basis that they stigmatised as much as threw any light on any unwelcome anomaly. See https://www.gcph.co.uk/latest/news/641_the_glasgow_effect_and_the_scottish_effect_unhelpful_terms_which_have_now_lost_their_meaning.

14. Mawson was consulted at the beginning of the government programme and again at the end, when he joined a firm tendered to stage a rescue package. But by that time it was 'too late' to save the programme he told government.

15. The Scottish body Arts in Healthcare was created out of an association with Paintings in Hospital in 2005. https://www.artinhealthcare.org.uk/about-history.php While in Northern Ireland, a mapping report was similarly carried out in 2001. http://www.artsandhealth.ie/about/a-history-of-arts-and-health-in-ireland/. A fuller account of the 'political background' of devolution is given in chapter three of Daisy Fancourt's book on designing Arts in Health interventions (Fancourt, 2017).

16. This plan subsequently "faltered through a change of minister" it is noted with frustration in the APPGAHW report (APPHAHW, 2017: 69).

17. So described because opposition to Labour government was traditionally seen as counterproductive. See this blog for details: https://www.iwa.wales/agenda/2021/09/review-the-welsh-way-essays-on-neoliberalism-and-devolution/.

18. See more info here: https://centreforpossiblestudies.wordpress.com/about/ and 'On the Edgeware Road': https://www.serpentinegalleries.org/whats-on/edgware-road/

19. Though not in Wales where its introduction was blocked by The Senedd.

20. See my PhD for an account of this relation (Williams, 2019: 43).

21. He bemoans how it was CEMA not ENSA that was taken as the model for the Arts Council of Great Britain. "We might wonder how differently the state's relationship with the arts might have been if the ENSA approach of working with popular culture had continued in peacetime" (ibid, p. 84).

22. https://www.england.nhs.uk/2016/02/health-as-a-social-movement/.

CHAPTER 5

Temporalities

In the introduction I set out my aim to examine the idea of creative health through an exploration of its genealogies, especially the histories of its former iteration as Arts in Health. This was a critical appraisal, I ventured at the outset, that would attempt to set mutable arts-health expressions within the political and economic contexts of their time and place. Interpretations of these histories, cited by advocates active in the field today, have also been included to show which have been claimed (or left unclaimed) as those that best represent the field's "roots" (White, 2009).

The choice to begin this study in the years before and after the Second World War was made on the understanding that the NHS has established the overarching institutional framework for this field of practice to be emerge and find recognition in the UK. This starting point was chosen in contrast to other historical accounts of Arts in Health that commonly locate origins much further back in prehistory, with the "beginning of art" itself (Fancourt, 2017). Less examined, I proposed, were thornier questions around how the metanarratives of our post-industrial, post-colonial, neoliberal age have informed the creation of the field of practice known as Arts in Health, especially across the UK's four nations.

In grappling with this sprawling task, I acknowledged at the outset the potential folly of using the word 'neoliberal' as catch-all criticism. Though

F. Williams, *When Was Arts in Health?*,
https://doi.org/10.1007/978-981-19-3617-3_5

"associated with a wider global transformation in politics, economics and everyday life", this descriptor requires interpretation in relation to specific fields, practices and sites (Davies et al., 2022: 2). Over the preceding chapters, multi-national perspectives have been charted, those which query the simple narrative that Arts in Health represents a social movement always able to promote positive social change regardless of the contexts or settings within which practitioners act.[1] Rather, I have tried to show how this assumption might obscure regressive devolutions as much as it drives progressive evolutions.

I will now conclude by tracing a broad contour across the post-war decades and between tiers of UK government, structural forces that together have provided the "pre-conditions" for the field of Arts in Health to become a distinctive "substance in history" (Diedrich, 2016). The extent to which this field of practice "constitutes a cohesive social movement remains a question of nuanced debate" (Daykin, 2019a: 10) it has been observed. But the construction of Arts in Health as a pressure group able to influence government policy can be held, I will conclude by arguing, within a 20 period: between the election of Tony Blair (in 1997) and Teresa May (in 2017).

The latter's snap election delayed the publication of the APPGAHW report and, to the surprise of many, came very close to delivering a Labour Party government that adhered to socialist values (under Jeremy Corbyn). The Labour Manifesto of 2017, *For the Many Not the Few,* offered opportunity for creative health to be promoted through what was named here as a battle cry: to "fight health inequalities" (Labour, 2017: 67).[2] But this opportunity was narrowly lost in 2017, and with it, the chance to align the argument for creative health with social democratic values and principles. From this point onward, new battle lines are drawn around culture, now enlisted in a populist 'culture war', with Donald Trump assuming power in the USA in same year as May clung on to her position as PM by a slim majority in the UK.

CHAPTER SUMMARY

In the preceding chapters, periods of economic boom and bust are shown to have shaped the relation of culture to health in ever-changing ways. The British Labour movement first grew amongst communities and cultures based in the industrial regions of the UK, those that flourished in Wales, Scotland and the North of England. Solidarities were forged through class alligance in The Great Depression of the 1930s, with trade unions fighting for worker's rights and improvements in living conditions. Mine workers found ways to collectively carry the risk of sickness and cost of healthcare (the Tredegar model), with Aneurin Beavan envisioning 'health' as a central plank of a holistic vision for a more egalitarian post-war society.

Gaining power through the landslide Labour victory in 1945, Bevan created the NHS at a time of national bankruptcy when the deprivations of wartime austerity were still being acutely felt. This achievement was made possible by the popular sense that some compensation and reward—for sacrifices made during the war—were now due. Bevan read the public mood of his day when he asked, "Why must the people wait any longer?", a question which acknowledged the extent and limit of human suffering. Within this temporal framing, preventative health was understood as "collective action" that might "build-up a system of social habits" that could create a fairer, more equal society.

The figure of the artist, however, could only be loosely associated with this hopeful project since "*some day* under the impulse of collective action", we shall "enfranchise the artists, by giving them our public buildings to work upon" (Bevan, 1952: 72 *my italics*). The idea that artists might craft social infrastructures, beyond those represented by public buildings, had not yet been articulated. Rather, artistic value was still judged by the "Modern art critic" who deferred to the needs of the "rich patron" (ibid, p. 72). The role of the artist in what were described by Jenny Lee, as "civilized communities", had yet to be found (Lee, 1965).

Unlike the Labour movement in Bevan's time, first wave social movements in the 1960s sprung-up not at a time of austerity, but economic growth. New expressions of counterculture were generational in their appeal. Complaint against the way in which biomedical power was exercised informed the demands of revolutionary movements, many of whom rejected pathology as a social harm: "stop treating homosexuality as an illness" (GLF, 1971). A "social hiatus" (Ingram, 2020: 3) enabled change to be enacted through forms of everyday life and new social relationships, not only the structural redistributions afforded by the welfare state. It has been more recently observed that they also, inadvertently or not, served to "undermine the structures and institutions of the welfare state by elaborating critiques of the paternalism, patriarchy, racism, sexism and ableism which were found in those institutions" (Davies et al., 2022: 14).

Tapping into international social movements, a new understanding of arts and culture's relation to health was advanced in the UK by way of community heath activists. Like other activist healthcare workers of this era (Dr Tudor Hart, nurse Elizabeth Anionwu), Dr Carl Clowes diagnosed a "wider prescription" for health than biomedicine alone could provide. 'Counter clinics' attempted to address the negative health impacts of racism amongst communities living in inner city areas across UK cities (Liverpool Black Sisters). The new figure of the Community Artist supported health activists to realise a vision of "cultural plurality" enabled by what was termed, "cultural democracy" (Kelly, 1984; Jeffers & Moriarty, 2017).

Operating across a range of community contexts, the artist in the 1970s and 80s became a "new kind of political activist" (Kelly, 1984: 12), one able to assist local health campaigns to protest the closure of local hospitals (Loraine Leeson). Artists secured 'placement' within the structure of The Hospital (Peter Senior) and sought to open-up critical space within corporations and government departments too (The Artist Placement Group). The late 1970s brought about a radical re-think of the premise on which the political economy was understood, with neoliberal ideology enthusiastically adopted by Margaret Thatcher through her Monetarist policies. In response, many activists found themselves attracted by a democratised Labour Party and the local authorities controlled by a resurgent Left. These municipal socialisms were perceived as a threat by Thatcher who quashed her political opponents through abolishing this tier of local government in key cities—cutting off the funding for proto-Arts in Health projects in the process such as those supported by the Greater London Council (GLC).

The Left's commitment to diverse cultural projects was attacked in the right-wing press, positioned as 'loony' when set alongside projections of free market' rationalities'. Local councils were renounced by a national Labour Party keen to win electoral success through its own temporal strategic twist: that of New Labour. The interregnum between the end of Thatcherism, and the new alternate route of Tony Blair's Third Way, offered ground on which the category of Arts in Health was first constructed in the late 1990s. This moment offered opportunity for the "stitching together our stories into a larger and more coherent narrative" it has been subsequently noted (Hebron, 2018).

The field's institutions were built in the shadow of widening social division and the harms inflicted on the health of working-class communities living in areas that became post-industrial wastelands. As a result of Acts of Devolution enacted in the late 90s, a National Network for Arts in Health was conceived solely as an English body. Variegated public-private institutions—such as the Bromley-By-Bow Health Centre—were amongst the first to "disregard" the provisions of the Welfare state "in favour of privately capitalised and mixed economy models of cultural and social organisation" (Philips, 2011: 36).

With critical attention solely trained on the "operation of the welfare state as opposed to the operation of the market", the state was "too easily be blamed for social hardships" while "unregulated free market capitalism" was left "off the hook" (Friedli, 2012: 3). Further diminishments of the local democratic state were facilitated by a decade of policies of austerity. This prompted doubt, amongst some working in the field of Arts in Health, that unequal stakeholders could strike a fair 'balance' between them. They spoke of "the difficulties of working in an uncertain statutory, voluntary hybrid environment in which morale is weakened and compromised by institutional uncertainty" (White, 2014: 4).

One art critic identified a process of empowerment not towards a 'big society' so much as "a massive transference of power from artists to institutions, from the grass roots to the establishment, and from community groups to highly professionalised and inter networked charitable organisations" (Quaintence, 2017). Writing in the same year as the APPGAHW report was published, Morgan Quaintance concluded that alliances forged between private and public bodies had created a "wider strategic culture that strengthens and reinforces the spread of new conservatism", one which actively "impedes progressive development" (ibid, p. 1).

Moreover, the types of partnerships and networks that facilitate Arts in Health initiatives prove opaque when cut adrift from the scrutiny afforded by local democratic state. Connections made by highly networked social entrepreneurs and charities have served to silence the sound of the proverbial 'bed pan' that Aneurin Bevan wished to hear echoing down Whitehall corridors. The latest government policy initiative, The Health and Social Care Bill (2022) will further enable "market deregulation at scale" it has been lamented (Pollock et al., 2021), a Bill "silent on public accountability mechanisms at a system level and at the non-statutory 'place' level" (ibid, p. 3).

ANALYSIS: THE LONG 90S?

This narrative above suggests that Arts in Health was produced out of specific set of social and economic conditions particular to the late 1990s. This is a decade that has subsequently been characterised by many as 'the long 90s', a period when "Left and right merged, state and economy were integrated in increasingly informal ways, and politics lost its fixed points" (Bang Larson, 2012: 1). The term has gained currency amongst broader accounts of how our sense of time has stalled, producing "lost futures" through the limitation of "capitalist realism" (Fisher, 2009). "It is easier to imagine the end of the world than the end of capitalism" (ibid, p. 2). "Neoliberal hegemony" has resulted in an ongoing sense, particularly felt amongst cultural producers, that "we have never left the epoc" of the 1990s (Gilbert, 2014, p. 5).

It was in the shadow of economic recession and the social conflict of the 1980s that Arts in Health emerged as a named entity, exploiting continuities enabled by Tony Blair's *Third Way*. This provided a way in which the Humanities in Healthcare (as the field then characterised itself) could be floated as a "bridgehead" between Labour and Conservative governments (Chamberlayne & Rupp, 2005). BBBHC modelled one of the first "integrated" Arts in Health spaces, enabling transgressive boundary crossings between the professional and amateur, the civic and the statutory, the profitable and the non-profitable. It piloted a type of hybrid institution whose "porous boundaries… allowed it to filter aspects of the welfare environment which would distort the way it works" (ibid, 107).

Integrated care, it has been noted recently, cannot provide a "miracle cure" to the problem of social and health inequality (Blumental, 2020). Rather, it depends on how institutional structures are navigated via their processual use over time (Burns et al., 2022). Yet the model of BBBHC continues to be championed in 2022 as a one through which community empowerment might be achieved for all people, living everywhere, regardless of its unique context and history (and indeed, ongoing use and development).[3] It has once again been appropriated as a model to be championed within the scope of the latest government policy initiative designed to address spatial inequality: that of 'levelling-up' (Johnson, 2022). "Organisations like the Bromley-by-Bow Centre (BBBHC) in East

London understand the importance of social infrastructure in helping to address inequalities" (Sansom, 2022).[4]

Mawson was able to trade on feelings of loss and disillusionment, so prevalent in the 1980s, to cast Liberal licence as "excess", a wasteful energy "mirrored in the culture of the public sector" (Mawson, 2008). His championing of the figure of the 'social entrepreneur' closed the gap between classic Liberal economics and more neoliberal conceptions of the public good—now made possible by market values integrated within healthcare, not *in spite of* them. His hybrid institution was able to find hopeful expression on the back of the lost faith in the "centralised, bureaucratic social democratic state", one which prompted social movements to argue "for devolved services shaped by, and run by and for, local people" (Davies et al., 2022: 14). This is precisely the premise and ambivalence upon which the negative characterisation of the NHS—made in the APPGAHW report—could be so undramatically staged, I would suggest.

The speculative analysis set out above suggests that Arts in Health can be seen as a social movement compatible with the adoption of neoliberal policies adopted across the health and cultural sectors—as much as it can and should be seen as one working in opposition to them. The growth and legitimisation of Arts in Health has been aided by the adoption of "neoliberal sensibilities" amongst civic actors (Boucher, 2019: 0). "The perceptions, feelings, ideas, and moral presuppositions—that underwrote how people conceived and encountered their world" (ibid, p. 1224).

Austerity has become a useful driver for creative innovation on terms that allow Arts in Health interventions to flourish, however reluctantly or enthusiastically exploited as such these opportunities might be. The creative impetus within healthcare can be placed within "the larger pattern through which an idea (of neoliberalism) is perceived, understood, felt, and experienced" (ibid, p. 1224). Beyond discrete aims of their own, those working Arts in Health are caught within institutional structures that have been relentlessly orientated towards private interest, felt by artists most of all, perhaps, as life-sapping "enstranglements" (Williams et al., 2022).

Lord Howarth appeared to acknowledge this entangled position when, in 2019, he proposed the idea of creative health as "a radical proposition, which one would expect to be uncongenial to neoliberal politicians" before adding: "Yet because of its demonstrable empirical validity it has been accepted by the Department of Health and the NHS" (Howarth, 2017: p. 1). Evidence-led policy has always necessitated the making of political choices and can be selectively applied by powerful interest groups who have proven themselves skilled practitioners of the art of politics as much as any that 'follows the science'. We can perhaps better observe this slippage from the viewpoint of 2022 since it is a distinction that has become more apparent during the period of the pandemic. In witnessing the role of medical advisors relative to politicians (Chris Witty to Boris Johnson, Anthony Fauci to Donald Trump), a clearer public understanding of the use and manipulation of scientific evidence has been made possible. This has always been the case, we can note, in relation to Michael Marmot's research and its relationship to certain policy choices—most notably that of austerity. Austerity has "hampered progress" in reducing inequality in the UK (BMA, 2016: 2), causing "excess death" well ahead of the pandemic (Toffolutti & Shurcke, 2019).

Danny Dorling and Kate Pikett wrote a critique of Marmot's work as early as 2010 where they queried his reticence to call for the rich to be taxed proportionately in more forthright terms. They detected timidity, not radicalism, in his report *Fair Society, Fair Lives*, characterising its recommendations as those "unlikely to frighten the horses" (Dorling & Pickett, 2010: p. 1231). They repeatedly point to "the lack of progress" in reducing inequality in the UK since The Black Report was published in 1980 (ibid, p. 1232). They continue to do so to this day in ever more direct terms: "Fall in life expectancy exposes 'levelling-up' *lies*...Turning the trends around will require real, not fake, commitment" (Dorling, 2021 *my emphasis)*. This is the "grim backcloth" behind the pandemic's latest stalling and reversal of mortality rates amongst certain UK populations, I suggest, the one against which Howarth's claim of "ground gained" falls so painfully short.

GROUND LOST

In Chap. 4, we left the narration of the development of Arts in Health at the point when the APPGAHW report was published, in 2017, three years before the pandemic broke out in spring 2020. I will now turn to chart some of the perceived progressions—and less heralded concessions—that have taken place over the last five years (2017–2022). I will emphasise the temporal use of place in the continuing iteration of creative health as "an idea whose time has come".

Firstly, we can note that selective adoptions of the APPGAHW report's recommendations were taken-up by the UK government under both May and Johnson's leadership. The referral mechanism of 'social prescription' (first tested by START in the 80s) was endorsed by Health Secretary Matt Hancock in 2018 who affirmed that "The arts and social activities" are "essential to our health and wellbeing" (Hancock, 2018).[5] They are also valuable for other "essential" financial reasons, he went on to state, as they can:

> help us move to more person-centred care and a focus on prevention as much as cure. Social prescribing can shape our health and social care system in the future... and help save money. (Hancock, 2018: 2)

As well as being warmly received by Secretary of State for Health on this cost-saving basis, the report also received "constructive criticism" on its political position from a practitioner within the field (of Art Therapy) who identified certain risks in the APPGAHW report's approach (Phillips, 2019). "The role of advocacy must be exercised with caution to avoid the accusation of producing propaganda" (ibid, p. 22), Kate Phillips warned. She further pointed to the underlying contradiction in positioning the arts as a force able to both "counter" as well as "complement" the medical model. She queried how "use of the arts" might extend into how the SDOH are currently understood:

> While the relationship between art, health and politics is not fully explored, the ethos of using the arts to address the social determinants of health is espoused, suggesting something *more fundamentally political* than a more humanised version of the current system. (ibid, p. 22, *my italics*)

As detailed in the last chapter, the APPGAHW reports quote Professor Richard Parish to provide a metaphor to explain how participating in creative activities might prevent ill-health. He characterises participation in the arts an "essential vaccine" in a wider "immunisation package" of "life skills" (APPGAHW, 2017: 30). Unerringly, this biomedical characterisation of the field was made just three years ahead of the global pandemic. This ill-fitting metaphor proffers a weak defence in the face of an ongoing global health crisis where vaccines underwrite our collective public health it could now be argued.

The power of the creative arts is held in the APPGAHW report as those that might "mitigate" the harmful social and health effects of inequality. Macroeconomic policies must be implemented to directly "eradicate" the causes of inequity, it is suggested (ibid, 29). This is a point so lightly made that the casual reader could be forgiven for missing it. But as previously underlined (in Chap. 4), it is a caveat that covers a rude truth: namely the failure to advance towards this goal by successive governments over the last 30 years. Social inequality has not shrunk to the point that it's causes might be "eradicated": inequality has dramatically ballooned since 2011.

There is now an "urgent need to do things differently, to build a society based on the principles of social justice" Michael Marmot concluded in 2021 identifying the "devastating intensity" with which inequality had been exacerbated post pandemic (Marmot et al., 2020). *The Build Back Fairer Covid-19* review notes that the UK has "fared badly" relative to other countries in its handling of the pandemic, with government "mismanagement" a "piece with what happened in England in the decade from 2010" over a decade of austerity (ibid, p. 5). Does this damning analysis of the government's inadequate response to the pandemic plausibly point to Arts in Health as an idea whose time has passed and been left unfulfilled as much as one whose time has come?

At best, the contingent position adopted in 2017—the arts as a protective mitigation or vaccination against ill-health—suggests that the field of Arts in Health occupies a holding pattern or 'meanwhile' temporal space. Any larger realisation of these ambitions would require waiting for a radical new government. Or else continuing to press the existing one to act on its previous and current commitments—to address the 'burning injustice' of inequality (May, 2017) by 'levelling-up' (Johnson, 2022).

> this government is getting on with the job of uniting and levelling up the country. Access to good healthcare, a good education, skilled work, reliable transport – none of this should depend on where you live. We're changing the rules of the game to put fairness back at the heart of the system. (Johnson, 2022)

Since the election of Johnson in 2019, both implicit and explicit connections have been drawn to link this 'levelling-up' agenda and that of creative health. Implicit continuity can be found through how George Osborne framed Greater Manchester as a "counter-weight" to London (Osborne, 2015). Inequality continues to be cast by in spatial terms, using metaphors of balance, weighting and leverage. Such guiding metaphors suggests that levers of redress might be pulled to allow the wealth created in The North of England to match that generated in The South. Indeed, it was an image of military comradeship—rather than capitalist competition—that George Osborne used to insist that The North would "not rival The South", so much as "be its brother in arms as we fight for Britain's share of the global economy" (Osborne, 2015).

THE (MIS)PLACING OF THE NORTH

A sense of national unity is secured through pitching the UK against the rest of the world, with global trade recast as economic warfare. Post Brexit, the idea of Britain taking on a global trade role outside of the EU was described by civil servants as 'Empire 2.00'.[6] This term has subsequently been dismissed as a "neo-colonial fantasy" that profoundly misperceives the power the UK is able to exert in the world today, historian David Olusoga objects (Olusoga, 2017). Rather it represents "a nostalgic yearning for lost colonies—and the wealth and global influence that came with them" (ibid, 1).

Within the current political discourse of 'levelling-up', there has been little or no acknowledgement of "social gradient" as key to how health inequality in the UK might be addressed. This would require taxation proportionate to wealth across the whole of the population as well as the taxing of multi-national corporations who currently pay no or little tax in the UK. "The problem of health inequality within countries is the social gradient—from top to bottom, the lower our social position the worse our health" (Marmot, 2017: 29). An acute analysis is offered by an economist who identifies Johnson's 'levelling-up' agenda as an expedient political slogan that can usefully misrepresent both the nature of inequality by reference to the Thatcherite past:

> It does not address the inequality of 1 per cent. The North South rhetoric is 1980s and diversionary. This is not North versus South. It's one per cent versus the 99 per cent. It's the haves and havenots. It's shareholders versus workers. (McInroy, 2022)

Greater Manchester and 'The North' continue to provide the nexus through which many of the live political discourses around health inequality, clash and comingle. Nuanced, interpretations of the "place of place" in relation to culture and health have been proposed by researchers based in the North of England (Gilmore, 2013). Most recently, an explicit demand was made for culture to be "embedded in the government's levelling-up agenda" from a new APPG, the *Northern Culture All Party Parliamentary Group*. Health and culture are "inextricably linked" it is stated in this 2022 report titled *The Case for Culture*. Cultural policy is promoted as "possibly the quickest and also the most underused lever for levelling-up" (Shaw et al., 2022: 9). This proposal was pitched on this temporal basis, with culture cast as an accelerant'.[7]

As we have seen, further back in time, Manchester was the first city to set up a dedicated national body for *Arts For Health* in 1985 (Chap. 3). The arts have long been heralded here as a "social movement" linked to global social movements for justice (Senior, 1993). "We will nurture local activity that embraces a world view" (Parkinson, 2011). These commitments were declared ahead of the deal struck between GM city leaders and George Osborne in 2015, one which saw Global Britain championed through a different set of solidarities, those that could unite the North and the South of the UK *against* the rest of the world.

Regional devolution, though harbouring potential to offer local autonomy, was tied closely to policies of austerity, enabled by local political elites. Budgetary controls were made conditional on budget reduction, with financial support for transformational change granted over a slim five-year period by Westminster. This tight window of opportunity for 'system change' demanded an exacting "speed of approach" the former *Chief Officer of the Greater Manchester Health and Social Care Partnership* conceded in 2017. "Have we gone too quickly or not quickly enough? If I had my time again I think I would have phased the work more than we did" (Vize, 2015: 360). His words suggest that more time might be needed to enact change, should funding allow, over any quick result able to be won by way of cultural policy.

A sceptical view of culture as an accelerant for addressing regional inequality is further supported by a group of researchers whose findings show how arts funding systems can themselves *reproduce* inequalities as much as *mitigate* them. They identify the "potential reproduction of structural, place-based inequalities", those that have been "entrenched by the longer-term impacts of austerity" (Gilmore et al., 2021).[8] There is a need to reduce "inequality *within* the Greater Manchester region" across the city's ten boroughs, to perceive inequalities beyond those crudely drawn—by political actors for electoral gain—between The North and The South (Williams, 2019).[9]

Inequalities abound within Greater Manchester. The high-rise centre—if not the outer boroughs of Manchester—has become an emblem of rentier capitalism as continuing 'development' unfolds here alongside a deepening housing crisis. In Manchester City's public spaces, amongst the shadows of its towering office and student accommodation blocks, can be found a variety of public art works, statues both old and new. One contemporary work has been identified as exemplifying how learning can "travel through time" (Higgins, 2017). Manchester, artist Phil Collins contests, provides a "meeting point" where the "birth of capitalism" first met forms of "organised resistance" by workers. As part of a performative enactment, he re-located a stone statue of Friedrich Engels in the city, making a film as he drove it on the back of a lorry from in its former home in the Ukraine.[10]

It was a mischievous repatriation. Engels wrote his famous study of *The Conditions of Working Class in England* while living in Manchester in the 1840s, at that time, the heart of the industrial revolution.[11] But Engels influence as one of the founders of the communist party (along with Karl Marx) was no-where publicly marked in the city, Collins keenly observed. The statue now sits outside the *Home* arts centre where it acts as provocation and anomaly amongst other celebrated statues of the Victorian age (such as William Gladstone, former Prime Minister and anti-abolitionist). Artist posters ironically celebrate the city using the nick name 'Manc Hatten' to describe the city and its rapid financialised growth, to comic effect. Statues have been printed in the most English of creative mediums: the tea towel (Fig. 5.1). Both of these statues—since the BLM protests of 2020—now inform debate around which might be 'maintained or explained' as reviews are made of the city's cultural emblems.

Other playful (art) gestures that draw on past histories have been made since the pandemic in relation to public health. The Whitworth Gallery created a public programme entitled *The Natural Cultural Health Service* (or NCHS) which encompassed "outdoor activities that promote good physical and mental wellbeing".[12] This name is an inventive re-branding that stages a newly conceived NHS an example of what on critic dubs a 'mockstitution' (Sholette, 2006). These are imitative, "phantom institutions" playfully invented by artists intending to "confront and intervene within the bureaucratic landscape of actual corporations, businesses, municipalities, and states" (ibid, 28).

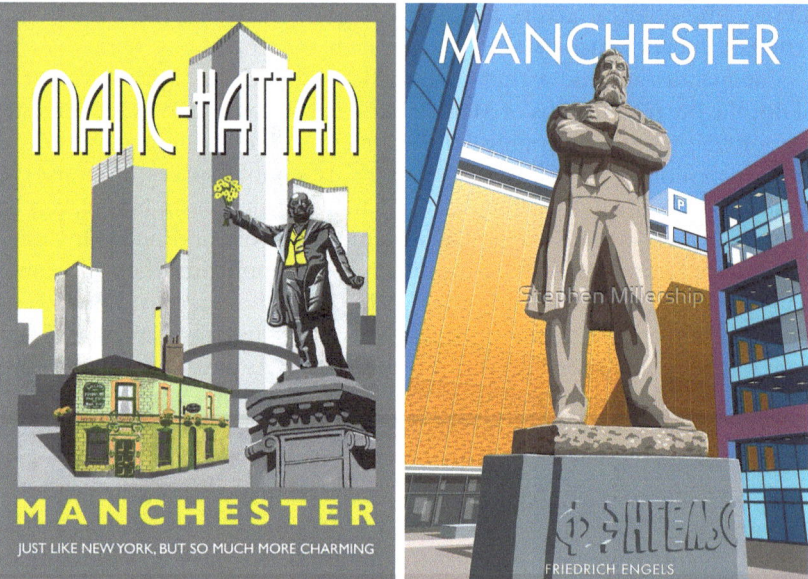

Fig. 5.1   Examples of how the City of Manchester ironically self-represents, by way of posters and tea towels adorned with its city statues

Whilst perhaps making for wry humour, the example of the NCHS surely takes on a different dimension when cited in The House of Lords as part of the tabling of an amendment to the 2020 Social and Health Care Bill. This bill was introduced to Parliament in 2021 to promote "more joined-up services and to ensure more of a focus on improving health rather than simply providing health care services" (Kings Fund, 2021). Lord Howarth used the example of the 'NCHS' to argue for the inclusion of a clause that would reference culture as a tool that could mitigate health inequality. It was cited amongst other Manchester-based case studies which all claimed to demonstrate the positive social impact of creative health since they were "targeted" at people living in the most "deprived areas" (Howarth, 2022).

Creative health is positioned here again as a possible accelerator to aid the "slow progress" on health inequality to date. Yet it is left unspecified as to which populations in the area around the Whitworth Gallery were deprived, relative to any other, and on what basis. It also leaves unexamined the reason behind the failures of cultural programmers to engage people living in deprived areas to date—as Howarth also notes that "those living in areas of higher deprivation are less likely to engage in them". The claim that "targeted investment in cultural and community opportunities" in deprived areas can mitigate health inequalities is difficult to uphold, without these qualifications, as a result.

The use of this fictitious example in a law-making context amply illustrates the risk, outlined above, of advocacy becoming a form of propaganda. This bunching together of different case studies, I would argue, leans all too heavily into desired outcomes at the expense of having to acknowledge difficulty, and contradiction, unevenness and nuance. Indeed, such a play on words could be perceived as a knowing misrepresentation—one that in turn could feed into broader perceptions of politicians as unreliable actors—those who present a "progressive veneer"[13] while part of an harmful "neoliberal consensus" (Evans et al., 2021: 5)

WORKPLACE SETTINGS

Nowhere is the gap between political rhetoric and social reality experienced more painfully perhaps than through the allocations of responsibility accorded to the figure of the 'the artist' working across local health and community settings. It is upon on this figure that so much of the responsibility for (policy) success is placed yet so little resource allocated or autonomy granted. Artists have seen a huge reduction in the real value of their incomes over the last ten years 2022, whilst being cast as both the villains and heroes of neoliberal ideology—champions of individualistic enterprise and as well as convenors of 'the social' (Jones, 2019; Pritchard, 2020).

It is towards a deeper understanding of the working conditions of creative (health) practitioners that important new critiques have emerged within the field over the last few years. These challenge the basis on which the field can be imagined to be sustainable in the future, demanding the acknowledgment that creative practitioners must themselves live well in order to "practice well" (Naismith, 2019). Nicola Naismith emphasises the need to address how inequalities are reproduced within the arts sector, proposing more support through structural reforms, not merely programmes offering self-care. Mike White's speculation of the "probable damnation" of the field finds form in Eleonor Belfiore's call for "fresh thinking on the *moral economy* of the subsidised arts sector", one that starts "from an acknowledgement that the normative environments of contemporary arts funding point to a clear moral failure" (Belfiore, 2022). "Embedded exploitation" is identified here "within the very fabric of the public infrastructure" (ibid, 18).

Other researchers constructively point to "resistance within an emerging movement" over how the arts now fit all too snugly within current medical treatment models. Yeoli et al. explore how artists operating as practitioners in healthcare contexts have "responded to the political and economic and policy transitions of recent years" (Yoeli et al., 2020). They return to the critiques of medicine mounted in the 1960s (outlined in Chap. 3) to identify how empowerment might be enabled through the "artistic gaze" over that of the "medical gaze". An artist focus provides human "dignity" when set alongside:

> the uni-directional power exerted by Foucault's concept of the *medical gaze* (Foucault, 1973) and is central to what renders Arts and Health so empowering. Participants value the gaze of the artist which, unlike that of the therapist, regards them as people with potential – potential to create, to inspire, to develop – rather than a problem to solve. (Raw et al., 2012)

They further warn of "potential negative outcomes" when considering the field's success in "normalizing" art practice within health care structures designed to improve health outcomes through cost savings. Forced to "align themselves more effectively with a 'treatment' model in order to access increasingly scarce funding resources," arts practitioners risk the loss of "the very value that their unique position as artists within the health care context confers" (Yoeli et al., 2020, p. 8).

I have offered my own reflection on the status of the artist as 'misfit' within Arts in Health settings. In a paper co-written with two artists (Becky Shaw and Anthony Schrag), we locate potentials for positive change within "hidden spaces close at hand within the institution" (ibid, p. 12). Unlike Daykin and Yeoli, the theories of space we propose are not predicated on the affordance of any 'boundary' (Daykin, 2019b; Yeoli et al., 2019). Rather than identify any outside "exo-space", we pose the possibility of the Arts in Health space as a temporal event, one 'whereby entrances and exists produce 'settings' for the production and recognition of arts-health knowledge. "The performance 'space' in which Arts in health practitioners 'act' is in this way utterly responsive to, and dependent upon, the conditions that generated them". Arts and Health practices do not take place within:

> some weightless, abstract nowhere, but are shaped by heavily weighed… histories and sets of agendas that are performed within particular social and political contexts. This institutional frame is rarely appraised or acknowledged in Arts in Health research. (Williams et al., 2022)

The least appraised frameworks are, perhaps, those institutional contexts constituted on behalf of creative health itself. Unlike the membership body of CHWA, the nation strategic body of the NCCH has extended its remit to work in partnership with the 'home nations'. While researchers now work within "integrated care systems" to explore "health at a systems level" in England, the NCCH also "works with colleagues in Northern Ireland, Scotland and Wales to share learning from the different systems and policy environments in the four nations".

Rather than acknowledge the weight of history, especially recent political history, these latest research sites have been portrayed by the new Director of the NCCH as virgin territory to be "discovered".[14] Places in the UK are said to present a "blank canvas" on which the positive effects of creative arts' integration into healthcare pathways might be measured. "In a way we're starting with a blank canvas, saying what is the problem and how can we respond to it together". Research studies set across different areas the UK, it is claimed, will help identify "the right conditions for this kind of work to flourish", with "knotty problems" with difficult "knots" eased through local co-production undertaken by local actors.[15]

> The translation of learning and how knowledge can be taken up elsewhere is not always obvious… Different regions have varied and "knotty" problems and that solutions must come from a place of co-production locally.

This learning approach upholds the possibility of 'scaling-up' whilst failing to acknowledge the specific political and economic conditions that both produce—and erase—the local. It risks a wilful ignorance of the conditions of history that constitute how creative healthy places come about—through contentious conflict and struggle as much as 'co-production'. Future research into the role of culture in relation to place could usefully recognise that "the objectives of researchers and policy makers are different" and that there is much to be gained from all parties understanding "how research-based evaluation might acknowledge, and learn from, failure and disagreement" (Atkinson et al., 2022). Deeper engagements with Human Geography could also inform how 'places' are understood and defined and the limitation of taking at face value pre-determined terms, such as 'levelling-up'. "To date the North has too readily followed deeply flawed processes (i.e., devolution deals) and embraced political slogans" (McEnroy, 2022) with the "problem of uneven development" persistently not "adequately defined and attended to" (Leyshon, 2021).

IMPLICATIONS FOR FUTURE RESEARCH

If the SDOH continue to underwrite the basis for this field of practice, then other theories of space and place in relation to inequality and culture will need to be utilised beyond that of 'levelling-up' alone. Post-pandemic, these could involve looking at the affordance of social space online: "Zoom is not a non-space" (Cowan et al., 2022) or the ethics of place within narratives of "displacement"—those that might inform more "mindful forms of 'placing'" (Adey et al., 2020). It might also further interrogate the types of methodological issues around research into health inequality, extending beyond the epidemiological, to re-examine causality in relation to "political systems" (Kelly-Irving et al., 2022). Or it could "more explicitly and widely apply an intersectional lens" into research into health inequalities especially those identified by way of place (Bambra, 2022: 1353).

Relevant to the pursuit of new research directions is the health of critique itself, which also occurs within specific contexts of time and place. Didier Fassin asks a doctorly question in his anthology *A Time for Critique* (Fassin, 2020): 'How is critique?' He references the recent closure of "departments in the humanities, the repeated targeting of the social sciences by representatives for their alleged lack of benefit for national economic interest" (Fassin, 2020: 22). "Substantial budget cuts for public research" are likely in the future, he speculates, since research "might undermine industrial companies by revealing their impact on health or climate". He points to those who regard critical thinking "as useless for markets, irrelevant for science, and, on the whole, potentially negative for the nation" (ibid, 22).

Fassin speculates that (economic) rationales provide "the most effective way of containing critique" without censoring it, since it can be allowed to develop "freely in as much as it does not overflow into society or contaminate positive science" (ibid, 23). Since these words were written, many arts and humanities departments have been dismantled across British Universities post-pandemic—by way of restructurings that trade union leaders condemn as politically motivated: "We have to see the attack on the arts as an attack on free speech".[16]

The ill-health of critique extends beyond the academy into popular—and populist—cultures. As Judith Butler and others have written on this point, public feeling is being galvanised against all types of intellectual discourse by resurgent social movements of the Alt Right. These seek to re-position the terms on which any rational public debate might be conducted (Butler, 2021), only emotive feelings and "nervous states" stirred (Davies, 2019). Such groups encourage the nation state "to intervene in university programs, to censor art and…threaten violence against immigrants", all moves designed to "restore a national order under duress" (Butler, 2021). Emotional attachment and loyalties to place are currently being secured through framing solidarities as those which bind us *against* others through metaphors of war.

This repressive trend responds to the awareness that the pandemic has provoked amongst publics of how our collective health depends on collective action in fundamental ways; through the support of key workers; inter-personal relationships, as well as through our wider relationship to the natural world. Understandings of this mutuality find expression in the slogan 'No one's health without everyone's' health', an affirmation informed by awareness of the risks posed not only by covid-19, but climate change too. Environmental health has prompted healthcare workers to ask what kind of "rapid responses" are ethical and demanded in the face of this global emergency—one that threatens all forms of liveable life on the planet (Salas, 2020).

Given the current the reassertion of nationalist narratives, Mike White's former characterisation of the field of Arts in Health as a "small scale global phenomenon" requires reappraisal, I would suggest. In an account written in 2009, White places a village in South Africa "at the epicentre" of the AIDS epidemic and the place where he begins the "story so far" of

Arts in Health. White says how on visiting one remote settlement, he felt like he had "journeyed to the interior of arts in health practice" (ibid, p. 11). This was because "although this is a place of sickness and poverty, there is also hope in the evident signs of a revitalized cultural tradition linked to health awareness".

Delegates from the Global South—South Africa specifically—were able to speak to this idea afresh through *The International Conference for Arts in Health* held online in 2021 (organised by CHWA). Unlike previous years, when this event was held in the city of Bristol, the new conference format enabled delegates to attend online. Delegates from over 30 countries spoke to the related topics of 'inequality, power and sustainability'. Alongside Lord Howarth's keynote speech—and some UK speakers who claimed that their efforts placed them "ahead of the pack" in a "world beating" position—was one delivered by Professor Pascale Allotey.[17] She explored the role of culture in codifying and reproducing inequality. She urged those listening to refuse the lure of easy emblems of nationalist pride in favour of promoting "art forms that throw into doubt who we are, how we engage with one another and how we engage with the planet".

Other delegates, speaking across various time zones, took up her call to use culture to question assumptions around the benevolence of culture and the social hierarchies that so often underwrite these.[18] Class division runs as deep in British culture, as it does in through the caste system in India, it was dryly noted. Such class distinctions are so naturalised over time that "no-one questions them" (Pradeep Narayanan). "Indigenous cultures" were discussed in relation to the need to "shed western concepts of well-being" (Patricia Navas). The importance of political agency was also underlined, especially the agency to "define culture and well-being on your own terms" (Chao Tatiana Main). These delegates brought perspectives that made them well-placed to judge the extent to which creative health is an idea whose time had come as they worked "between different spaces, timelines and understandings of the world" (Cowan et al., 2022).

In charting the currents on which Arts in Health has been floated as an 'idea' and practice, past and present, I have tried to plot points by which any further structural study of this shifting field might be made more possible. Genealogical study can help us "disentangle the conditions of (its) history from the density of discourse" (Foucault, xix). A wider, more open debate on the structural formation of this field, its national institutions and foundational values, is necessary beyond any afforded by an all-party parliamentary status quo. Less opaque, more democratic forms of decision-making would serve a broader range of interests and could inform how strategies for the future could be more collectively imagined by those working across intersectional social movements today. New groupings—such as *Lesbians and Gays Support the Migrants*—self-consciously echo solidarities forged in the past, reflecting the need for new alliances that respond to the multiple challenges of the current moment, especially those needed to counter hateful ideologies that trade on 'othering'. Histories of social movements exist as latent potentials for creative health and how it might be configured and understood in the present and the future. Intersectional inequalities in health can inform place-based understandings of the social determinants of health (Bambra, 2022).

Perhaps the comments by the conference delegates cited above prove that healthy critical discourses on how arts and culture might create health are already underway in other time zones and places apart from the UK, less audible or foregrounded, rather than simply absent. Such a hope aligns with the need to better and more fully understand "shared histories that have configured out present, in order to find more expansive and generous solutions to the problems we face" (Bhambra, 2021:14). Knowledge sharing calls forth its own "process of re-ordering" (Cowan et al., 2022: 1467). This is a call for material and environmental justice, yes, but one that demands epistemic justice too.

Notes

1. The focus has been on two nations within the UK (England and Wales, and to lesser extent, Scotland and Ireland). But also encompassing influences from France and America, with the direct support of the NHS given by people from Indian subcontinent and former commonwealth Caribbean nations.

2. Indeed, this was the very point that May chose to echo in her first speech which also talked of the "burning injustice" of health inequality, using language resonant of Aneurin Bevan's own description of it as a "burning luminous mark of interrogation" (Bevan, 1952: 1).

3. This continues to evolve and diverge from its original conception as much as building on it. See Lynne Froggett's account of the years following the departure of Andrew Mawson which brings to life the misgivings of staff held around various aspects of his approach.

4. This policy officer goes on to use this local example to advance the wider proposal that: "to get the best results from levelling-up investment, the government should listen to the growing chorus of people calling for greater devolution of power".

5. Hancock did not foreground the social determinants of health as part of how he saw this referral mechanism might better enable 'person-centred' healthcare.
6. For details of this story, read how the term came about and in what context here: https://www.civilserviceworld.com/professions/article/liam-fox-tells-civil-servants-not-to-use-offensive-term-empire-20.
7. Read about this initiative here: https://www.gmhsc.org.uk/opinion/greater-manchester-is-a-marmot-city-region-what-does-that-mean-and-how-will-it-improve-our-health-and-reduce-inequalities   Greater Manchester and Michael Marmot's Institute of Health Equity agreed a collaboration and programme of work for 2019–20 that saw Greater Manchester become a Marmot City Region. See https://www.instituteof-healthequity.org/about-our-work/latest-updates-from-the-institute/greater-manchester-a-marmot-city-region.
8. Read a summary in this blog. https://www.pec.ac.uk/blog/when-policy-meets-place.
9. https://www.miahsc.com/news-2/2019/5/22/facing-inwards-and-outwards-challenging-inequalities-within-greater-manchester.
10. I wrote this section before the outbreak of war in the Ukraine in March 2022, when some people suggested the statue of Engels should be removed. Seehttps://www.newstatesman.com/comment/2022/03/tearing-down-the-statue-of-friedrich-engels-wont-help-ukraine.
11. Engels book was published in 1845. An English translation was published in 1885.
12. https://www.whitworth.manchester.ac.uk/whats-on/events/naturalcultural/.
13. Lord Howarth has indicated that this is precisely what Keir Starmer is considering in his attempt to emulate Welsh Labour's 'success'. See: https://nation.cymru/news/english-labour-party-needed-to-emulate-welsh-labours-success-says-report/.
14. Acting Director, Alexandra Coulter, speaking to Arts Professional in 2021: https://www.artsprofessional.co.uk/news/national-centre-creative-health-mainstream-arts-health-and-social-care. The use of the word "discovered" here echoes how Carmen Moersch characterised Gallery Education, as a territory mistakenly claimed by curators of the education turn as new territory: much as "Columbus 'discovered' America". See Chapter 4, section titled Culture Vultures.
15. The leader of the University and College Union, Jo O'Grady, quoted here: https://socialistworker.co.uk/news/roehampton-university-job-cuts/.

16. Elsewhere, in a more academic context, more sustained attention has been given to issues of power in relation to local place by Alex Coulter and Julia Fortier, I acknowledge (Fortier & Coulter, 2021).
17. Phil George, Chairman of Arts Council Wales, proposed Wales as being 'ahead of the pack' by way of the 'world beating' policy framework provided by the Future Generations Act. See https://wahwn.cymru/2021/06/In-the-Zones/. Pascale Allotey is the public health researcher and the Director of the United Nations University International Institute for Global Health.
18. Named in programme: https://www.artshealthresources.org.uk/docs/culture-health-wellbeing-conference-report/.

REFERENCES

Acheson, D. (1997). Independent inquiry into inequalities in health. https://
assets.publishing.service.gov.uk/government/uploads/system/uploads/
attachment_data/file/265503/ih.pdf

Adamson, E. (1984). *Art as healing: Edward Adamson.* The Adamson Collection.

Addae, P., & Danquah, S. (2021). *Health activism in Brixton.* Centric Community
Research. https://centric.org.uk/blog/health-activism-in-brixton

Adey, P., Bowstead, J., Brickell, K., Desai, V., Dolton, M., Pinkerton, A., & Siddiq,
A. (2020). *The handbook of displacement.* Palgrave Macmillan. https://doi.
org/10.1007/978-3-030-47178-1

Allen, F. (2008). Situating gallery education. *Tate Encounters.* https://www.tate.
org.uk/tate-encounters/edition2/tateencounters2_felicity_allen.pdf

Allen, J. (2012). 1938: The Finsbury Park Health Centre. The 20th Century
Society. Retrieved from https://c20society.org.uk/100-buildings/1938-
finsbury-health-centre-london

All-Party Parliamentary Group on Arts Health and Wellbeing. (2017). *Creative
health: The arts for health and wellbeing* (2nd ed.). AAPG. Retrieved from
http://www.artshealthandwellbeing.org.uk/APPG-inquiry/Publications/
Creative_Health_Inquiry_Report_2017_Second_Edition.pdf

Anderson, W. (1998, Fall). Where is the postcolonial history of medicine? *Review
in the Bulletin of the History of Medicine, 72*(3), 522–530.

Antonovsky, A. (1979). *Health, stress, and coping.* Jossey-Bass.

Arts Council England Health Development Agency. (2000). Art for health: A
review of good practice. https://assets.publishing.service.gov.uk/govern-
ment/uploads/system/uploads/attachment_data/file/142883/Art_for_
Health.pdf

© The Author(s), under exclusive license to Springer Nature
Singapore Pte Ltd. 2023   127
F. Williams, *When Was Arts in Health?,*
https://doi.org/10.1007/978-981-19-3617-3

Arts Council Wales. (2009). Arts in health and wellbeing: An action plan for Wales. http://www.artshealthresources.org.uk/wp-content/uploads/2017/02/2009-Arts-in-Health-and-Well-Being-An-Action-Plan-for-Wales.pdf

Arts Council Wales. (2018). *Arts and health in Wales: A mapping study of current activity. Volume 1: Analysis, findings and proposals.* Arts Council of Wales.

Arts Council of Wales and Welsh Assembly Government. (2009). *Arts in health and wellbeing: An action plan for Wales.* Arts Council of Wales.

Arts for Health. (2012). *Art and health manifesto part 2.* Manchester Metropolitan University. http://www.artshealthresources.org.uk/docs/arts-andhealth-manifesto-part-2/

Atkinson, S., Evans, B., Woods, A., & Kearns, R. (2015). The 'medical' and 'health' in critical medical humanities. *Journal of Medical Humanities, 36,* 71–81.

Atkinson, S., MacNaughton, J., & Richards, J. (Eds.). (2016a). *The Edinburgh companion to the critical medical humanities.* Edinburgh University Press. http://www.jstor.org/stable/10.3366/j.cttlbgzddd

Atkinson, S., Macnaughton, J., & Richards, J. (Eds.). (2016b). Introduction. In *The Edinburgh companion to the critical medical humanities* (pp. 1–32). Edinburgh University Press. http://www.jstor.org/stable/10.3366/j.cttlbgzddd.5.

Atkinson, D., Bianchini, F., Burgess, G., & Oanca, A. (2022, May). Evaluating cities and capitals of culture. *Arts Professional.* https://www.artsprofessional.co.uk/magazine/article/evaluating-cities-and-capitals-culture

Ayo, N. (2012). Understanding health promotion in a neoliberal climate and the making of health conscious citizens. *Critical Public Health, 22*(1), 99–105. https://doi.org/10.1080/09581596.2010.520692

Bachrach, L. L. (1978). A conceptual approach to deinstitutionalization. *Hospital and Community Psychiatry, 29*(9), 573–578.

Baggs, C. (2003). 'The whole tragedy of leisure in penury': The South Wales miners' institute libraries during the great depression. *Libraries and Culture, 39*(2), 115–136.

Bambra, C. (2022). Placing intersectional inequalities in health. *Health and Place, 75,* 1353–8292.

Bambra, C., & Schrecker, T. (2015). *How politics makes us sick: Neoliberal epidemics.* Palgrave Macmillan.

Bang Larson, L. (2012). The Long Nineties: Revisiting art's social turn and the 1990s: the decade that has yet to end. *Frieze, 144.* https://www.frieze.com/article/long-nineties

Banner, O. (2017). *Communicative biocapitalism: The voice of the patient in digital health and the health humanities.* University of Michigan Press.

Bates, V., Goodman, S., & Bleakley, A. (Eds.). (2014). *Medicine, health and the arts: Approaches to the medical humanities.* Routledge.

Belfiore, E. (2006). The social impacts of the arts – myth or reality? In M. Mirza (Ed.), *Culture vultures* (pp. 20–37) Policy Exchange. https://www.policyexchange.org.uk/wp-content/uploads/2016/09/culture-vultures-jan-06.pdf

Belfiore, E. (2022). Who cares? At what price? The hidden costs of socially engaged arts labour and the moral failure of cultural policy. *European Journal of Cultural Studies, 25*(1), 61–78. https://doi.org/10.1177/1367549420982863

Bell, S. E. (2002). Jo Spence's narratives of living with illness. *Health: An Interdisciplinary Journal for the Social Study of Health, Illness and Medicine, 6*(1), 5–30.

Bell, K., & Green, J. (2016). On the perils of invoking neoliberalism in public health critique. *Critical Public Health, 26*(3), 239–243. https://doi.org/1 0.1080/09581596.2016.1144872

Berger, J. (1972). *Ways of seeing*. Penguin.

Berridge, V. (1999). The Black Report. As archived on Socialist Health Association website: https://www.sochealth.co.uk/national-health-service/public-health-and-wellbeing/poverty-and-inequality/the-black-report-1980/the-origin-of-the-black-report/interpreting-the-black-report/

Bevan, A. (1940, June 21). *Tribune*.

Bevan, A. (1945). We are the builders. In an election speech of 1945. https://spartacus-educational.com/TUbevan.htm

Bevan, A. (1946). Bevan's speech on the Second reading of the NHS Bill 30 April 1946. *House of Commons*. https://www.sochealth.co.uk/national-healthservice/the-sma-and-the-foundation-of-the-national-health-service-dr-leslie-hilliard-1980/aneurin-bevan-and-the-foundation-of-the-nhs/bevans-speech-on-the-second-reading-of-the-nhs-bill-30-april-1946/

Bevan, A. (1948, July 2). July 5th and the socialist advance. *Tribune*, 7.

Bevan, A. (1950, February 3). The people's coming of age. *Tribune*, 14.

Bevan, A. (1952). *In place of fear*. Quartet Books.

Bevan, A. (1956). *In place of fear*. Heinemann.

Bevan, A. (1958, November 21). Independence – Then hard work: How to maintain the frontiers of liberty. *Tribune*, 5.

Beveridge, W. H. B. (1942). *Social insurance and allied services: Report by Sir William Beveridge*. H.M. Government.

Bhambra, G. (2021). Relations of extraction, relations of redistribution: Empire, nation, and the construction of the British welfare state. *British Journal of Sociology, 73*(1), 4–15.

Bhattacharyya, G., Elliott-Cooper, A., Balani, S., Nisanciouglu, K., Koram, K., Gebrial, D., El-Enany, N., & De Noronha, L. (2020). *Empire' endgame: Racism and the British state*. Pluto Press.

Bishop, C. (2010). *Rate of return: The artist placement group*. Artforum. October Issue.

Biven, R. (2015). *Contagious communities, medicine, migration and the NHS in post-war Britain*. Oxford University Press.

Bivens, R., & Crane, R. (2017). What is the N in the NHS? In H. Quilter-Pinner & M. Gorsky (Eds.), *Devo-Then, Devo-Now: What can the history of the NHS tell us about localism and devolution in health and care?* Institute of Public research.

Blair, T. (1997). Leader's speech, party conference, Brighton. http://www.britishpoliticalspeech.org/speech-archive.htm?speech=203

Blair, T. (1999a). The class war is over. Speech to the labour party conference. http://www.britishpoliticalspeech.org/speech-archive.htm?speech=205

Blair, T. (1999b). Leader's speech, party conference, Bournmouth. http://www.britishpoliticalspeech.org/speech-archive.htm?speech=205

Blair, T. (2001). Launching labour's manifesto at Southampton University. https://www.theguardian.com/politics/2001/may/23/labour.tonyblair

Blair, T. (2013). My job was to build on some of Thatcher's Policies. *BBC news.* https://www.bbc.co.uk/news/av/uk-politics-22073434

Bleakley, A. (2014). Towards a 'critical medical humanities. In V. Bates, A. Bleakley, & S. Goodman (Eds.), *Medicine, health and the arts: Approaches to the medical humanities.* Routledge.

Blumberg, M. (1999). The AIDS Memorial Quilt as Performance: creating healing narratives. In D. Haldane & S. Loppert (Eds.), *The arts in healthcare: Learning from experience.* The Kings Fund.

Blumental, D. (2020). Making integration work. *Comparative Health Systems Performance, 55*, 3. https://onlinelibrary.wiley.com/doi/full/10.1111/1475-6773.13575

Boston Women's Health Collective. (1973). *Our bodies, our selves.* Women's Press.

Boucher, E. (2019, October). Anticipating Armageddon: Nuclear risk and the neoliberal sensibility in Thatcher's Britain. *The American Historical Review, 124*(4), 1221–1245. https://doi.org/10.1093/ahr/rhz744

Bourdieu, P. (1965). *Distinction: A social critique of the judgement of taste.* Routledge.

Bourdieu, P. (1984). *Distinction: A social critique of the judgement of taste.* Routledge and Kagan Paul Ltd.

Bridges, K., Keel, T., & Obasogie, O. (2017). Introduction: Critical race theory and the health sciences. *American Journal of Law and Medicine, 43*(2-3), 179–182.

British Medical Association. (2016). Health in all policies: health, austerity and welfare reform. A briefing from the board of science. https://www.bma.org.uk/media/2086/bos-health-in-all-policies-austerity-briefing-2016.pdf

Broderick, S. (2011). Arts practices in unreasonable doubt? Reflections on understandings of arts practices in healthcare contexts. *Arts Health, 3*(2), 95–109.

Brooks, S. (2017). *Why Wales never was: The failure of Welsh nationalism.* University of Wales Press.

Broughton, J. (2013). Municipal dreams. 'Noting is too good for ordinary people'. https://municipaldreams.wordpress.com/2013/04/09/finsbury-health-centre-nothing-is-too-good-for-ordinary-people/

Brown, L. (1993). *Art and soul and the cold blue walls: Writings about art*. Oldham Metropolitan Borough Council.

Brown, L. (2006). *Is art therapy? Art for mental health at the millennium*. Manchester Metropolitan University.

Broxton, A. (2017). "Why should the people wait any longer?" – How labour built the NHS. https://tidesofhistory.com/2017/07/05/why-should-the-people-wait-any-longer-how-labour-built-the-nhs/

Burns, H. (2015). Make the NHS a well-being service not sickness. *The New Scientist Magazine*. https://www.newscientist.com/article/dn27197-make-the-nhs-a-well-being-service-not-sickness-service/#ixzz7KHoKoGqp

Burns, L., Nembhard, I., & Shortell, S. (2022). Integrating network theory into the study of integrated healthcare. *Social Science and Medicine, 296*, 114664.

Burtenshaw, R. (2019). How the NHS was won. *Tribune Magazine*. https://tribunemag.co.uk/2019/07/how-the-nhs-was-won

Butler, J. (2009). Critique, dissent, disciplinarity. *Critical Inquiry, 35*, 773–795.

Butler, J (2021). Why is the idea of 'gender' provoking backlash the world over? *The Guardian*. Retrieved from https://www.theguardian.com/us-news/commentisfree/2021/oct/23/judith-butler-gender-ideology-backlash

Caduff, C. (2020). What went wrong: Corona and the world after the full stop. *Medical Anthropology Quarterly, 34*(4), 467–487.

Callard, F., & Fitzgerald, D. (2015). *Rethinking interdisciplinarity across the social sciences and neurosciences*. Palgrave Macmillan.

Cameron, D. (2010a). Transcript of a speech by the Prime Minister on the Big Society. https://www.gov.uk/government/speeches/big-society-speech

Cameron, D. (2010b). *Speech on wellbeing*. Cabinet Office. https://www.gov.uk/government/speeches/pm-speech-on-wellbeing

Camic, P., & Clift, S. (2016). *Oxford textbook of creative arts, health, and wellbeing. International perspectives*. Oxford.

Chamberlayne, P., & Rupp, S. (2005). 'Only connect': Report on the Bromley-by-Bow Project. SOSTRIS STAGE TWO AGENCY STUDY. https://www.uel.ac.uk/sites/default/files/7302.pdf

Chamberlayne, P., & Rupp, S. (2007). 'Only connect': Report on the Bromley-by-Bow Project. SOSTRIS STAGE TWO AGENCY STUDY. https://www.uel.ac.uk/sites/default/files/7302.pdf

Chandler, D., & Redi, J. (2016). *The neoliberal subject: Resilience, adaptation and vulnerability*. Rowman & Littlefield.

Chatterjee, H., & Noble, G. (2017). *Museums, health and well-being*. Routledge.

Chetty, D. (2022). *Welsh (plural) essay on the future of Wales*. Watkins Media.

Christie, Y., & Hill, N. (2003). *Black spaces project*. The Mental Health Foundation.

Clements, N. (2017). The pioneers and the Welsh community arts movement: A view from Wales. In *Culture, democracy and the right to make art: The British community arts movement* (pp. 99–114). Bloomsbury Collections.

Clements, D., Donald, A., Earnshaw, M., & Williams, A. (2008). *The future of community reports of a death greatly exaggerated*. Pluto Press.

Clift, S., & Camic, P. M. (2016). Introduction to the field of creative arts, wellbeing and health: Achievements and current challenges. In S. Clift & P. M. Camic (Eds.), *Oxford textbook of creative arts, health, and wellbeing. International perspectives on practice, policy, and research* (pp. 3–10). Oxford University Press.

Clift, S., Camic, P. M., Chapman, B., Clayton, G., Daykin, N., Eades, G., Parkinson, C., Secker, J., Stickley, T., & White, M. (2009). The state of arts and health in England. *Arts and Health, 1*(1), 6–35. https://doi.org/10.1080/17533010802528017

Clift, S., Philips, K., & Pritchard, S. (2021). The need for robust critique of research in arts and health. *Cultural Trends, 30*(5), 442–459.

Colgrove, J. (2002). The McKeown thesis: A historical controversy and its enduring influence. *American Journal of Public Health, 92*(5), 725–729. https://doi.org/10.2105/ajph.92.5.725

Conford, P. (2020). *Realising health: The Peckham experiment, its descendants and the spirit of Hygiea*. Cambridge Scholars Publishing.

Cosgrove, J. (2002, May). The McKeown thesis: A historical controversy and its enduring influence. *American Journal of Public Health, 92*(5), 725–729.

Coupland, N. (2008). Chapter 8. Aneurin Bevan, class wars and the styling of political antagonism. In P. Auer (Ed.), *Style and social identities* (pp. 213–246). De Gruyter Mouton. https://doi.org/10.1515/9783110198508.2.213

Cowan, H., Kühlbrandt, C., & Riazuddin, H. (2022). Reordering the machinery of participation with young people. *Sociology of Health and Illness.* https://doi.org/10.1111/1467-9566.13426

Crane, R., & Bivens, R. (2017). What is the N in the NHS? In H. Quilter-Pinner & M. Gorsky (Eds.), *Devo-Then, Devo-Now: What can the history of the NHS tell us about localism and devolution in health and care?* Institute of Public Research.

Crenshaw, K. (1991). Mapping the margins: Intersectionality, identity politics, and violence against women of color. *Stanford Law Review, 43*(6), 1241–1299.

Crossley, N. (1998). R.D. Laing and the British anti-psychiatry movement: A socio historical analysis. *Social Science and Medicine, 47*(7), 877–889.

Crossley, N. (2005). *Making sense of social movements*. Open University Press.

Cultural Policy Collective. (2004). *Beyond social inclusion. Towards cultural democracy*. Cultural Policy Collective.

D'Arcona, M. (2015). George Osborne's conference speech: ECHOES of Aneurin Bevan. https://www.theguardian.com/commentisfree/2015/oct/05/george-osborne-conference-speech-verdict-chancellor

Davies, W. (2019). *Nervous states. How feeling took over the world*. Vintage.

Davies, W. (2020). The Great British Battle: How the fight against coronavirus spread a new nationalism. *The Guardian.* https://www.theguardian.com/books/2020/may/16/the-great-british-battle-how-the-fight-against-coronavirus-spread-a-new-nationalism

Davies, W., & Gane, N. (2020). Post-neoliberalism? An introduction. *Theory, Culture and Society, 38*(6), 3–28. Retrieved from: https://www.theoryculturesociety.org/blog/special-issue-post-neoliberalism

Davies, C., Rosenberg, M., Knuiman, M., Ferguson, R., Pikora, T., & Slatter, N. (2012). Defining arts engagement for population-based health research: Art forms, activities and level of engagement. *Arts and Health: An International Journal for Research, Policy and Practice, 4*(3), 203–216.

Davies, A., Jackson, B., & Sutcliffe-Braithwaite, F. (2021). *The neoliberal age? Britain since the 1970s.* University College London.

Daykin, N. (2019a). *Arts, health and well-being: A critical perspective on research, policy and practice* (1st ed.). Routledge.

Daykin, N. (2019b). Social movements and boundary work in arts, health and wellbeing: A research agenda. *Nordic Journal of Arts, Culture and Health., 1*(1), 9–20.

Del Castillo, J., Khan, H., Nicholas, L., & Finnis, A. (2016). *Health as social movement, the power of people in movements.* NESTA. Retrieved from: https://www.nesta.org.uk/report/health-as-a-socialmovement-the-power-of-people-in-movements/

Della Porta, D., & Diani, M. (2010). *Social movements: An introduction* (2nd ed.). Blackwell.

Department of Health. (1999). *Saving lives: Our healthier nation.* Stationary Office. https://assets.publishing.service.gov.uk/government/uploads/system/uploads/attachment_data/file/265576/4386.pdf

Department of Health. (2007). A prospectus for arts and health. http://webarchive.nationalarchives.gov.uk

Diedrich, L. (2007). *Treatments, language, politics, and the culture of illness.* University of Minnesota Press.

Diedrich, L. (2016). *Indirect action: Schizophrenia, epilepsy, AIDS, and the course of health activism.* University of Minnesota Press.

Dorling, D. (2021). Grim fall in life expectancy exposes UK government's "levelling up" lies. *Open Democracy.* https://www.dannydorling.org/?page_id=8341

Dorling, D., & Pickett, K. (2010). Against the organization of misery? The Marmot review of health inequalities. *Social Science and Medicine, 71,* 1231–1233.

Dorling, D., Stuart B., & Stubbs, J., (2016). Brexit, inequality and the demographic divide. https://blogs.lse.ac.uk/politicsandpolicy/brexit-inequality-and-the-demographic-divide/

Dorman, F., Butcher, H., & Taunt, D. (2016). *Catalyst or distraction? The evolution of devolution in the English NHS.* The Health Foundation. ISBN 978-1-906461-78-2.

Dose, L. (2006). National network for the arts in health: Lessons learned from six years of work. *The Journal of the Royal Society for the Promotion of Health, 126*(3), 110–112.

Dowden, O. (2021). We won't allow Britain's history to be cancelled. *The Telegraph.* https://www.telegraph.co.uk/news/2021/05/15/wont-allow-britains-history-cancelled/

Ehrenreich, B., & Ehrenreich, J. (1978). *Medicine and social control. The cultural crisis of modern medicine* (pp. 39–79). Monthly Review Press.

El Gingihy, Y. (2017). *How to dismantle the NHS in 10 easy steps: The blueprint that the government does not want you to see.* Zero Books.

Engels, F. (2009). *The condition of the working class in England.* Penguin Classics.

Evans, T. (2022). Mapping the Welsh way. *International Socialism, A Quarterly Review of Socialist Theory* (174). Downloaded April 2022. http://isj.org.uk/welsh-way/

Evans, D., Smith, K., & Williams, H. (2021). *The Welsh way: Essays on neoliberalism and devolution.* Parthian.

Fancourt, D. (2017). *Arts in health. Designing and researching interventions.* Oxford University Press.

Fancourt, D. & Finn, S. (2019). *What is the evidence on the role of the arts in improving health and well-being? A scoping review.* WHO Regional Office for Europe (Health Evidence Network (HEN) synthesis report 67). http://www.euro.who.int/en/publications/abstracts/what-is-the-evidence-on-the-role-of-the-arts-in-improving-health-and-well-being-a-scopingreview-2019

Fanon, F. (1960). *The wretched of the earth.* First Black Cat Edition.

Farquharson, A. (2006, September) Bureaux de change. *Frieze* (101).

Fassin, D. (2020). How is critique? In D. Fassin & B. E. Hardcourt (Eds.), *A time for Critique.* Columbia University Press.

Fernando, S. (2005). Multicultural mental health services: Projects for minority ethnic communities in England. *Transcultural Psychiatry, 42,* 420–436.

Fisher, M. (2009). *Capitalist realism: Is there no alternative?* Zero Books.

Foucault, F. (1973). *The Birth of the Clinic: An Archaeology of Medical Perception.* Laing, R.D. (ed.) Routledge. London.

Foucault, M. (1976b). The will to knowledge: The history of sexuality, Volume 1 (trans. R. Hurley, 1998).

Foucault, M. (1997). *Society must be defended.* Picador.

Fox, D. (1985). Who we are: The political origins of the medical humanities. *Theoretical Medicine and Bioethics, 6,* 327–341.

Francis, H. (1976). The origins of the South Wales miners' library. *History Workshop, 2,* 183–205. Retrieved September 3, 2021, from http://www.jstor.org/stable/428807/

Friedli, L. (2012). 'What we've tried, hasn't worked': The politics of assets based public health. *Critical Public Health, 23*(2), 131–145. https://doi.org/1 0.1080/09581596.2012.748882

Froggett, L., & Chamberleyne, P. (2003). Bromley by Bow Centre research and evaluation project: Integrated pratice – Focus on older people.

Gay Liberation Front. (1971). Manifesto. Bishopsgate Archive. https://s3.eu-west-1.amazonaws.com/bishopsgate/GLF-Manifesto-1971.pdf?mtime= 20220707134248

Geddes, M. (2000). The modernization and improvement of government and public services: social exclusion—New language, new challenges for local authorities. *Public Money & Management, 20*(2), 55–60.

Genosko, G. (Ed.). (1996). *A Guttari reader.* Blackwell Publishers.

Gielen, P. (2013). *Institutional attitudes: Instituting art in a flat world.* Valiz.

Gielen, P. (Ed.). (2016). *Institutional attitudes: Instituting art in a flat world* (pp. 219–228). Valiz.

Gilbert, H., & Peck, H. (2014). *Service transformation: Lessons from mental health.* The Kings Fund.

Gilligan, A. (2012). The Olympic opening ceremony: A review. *The Telegraph.*

Gilmore, A. (2013). Cold spots, crap towns and cultural deserts: The role of place and geography in cultural participation and creative place-making. *Cultural Trends, 22*(2), 86–96.

Gilmore, A., Dunn, B., Barker, V., & Taylor, M. (2021). When policy meets levelling-up and the culture and creative industries. https://pec.ac.uk/blog/ when-policy-meets-place

Goffman, I. (1961). *Asylums: Essays on the social situation of mental patients and other inmates.* Doubleday.

Gould, S. (2018). Disorganisation/organisation: A response to a provocation by British Art Studies. In *British Art after Brexit.* https://www.britishartstudies. ac.uk/issues/issue-index/issue-20/british-art-after-brexit

Graeber, D., & Wengrow, D. (2021). *The dawn of everything: A new history of humanity.* Penguin.

Graham, J. (2014). *Para-sites like Us: What is this para-sitic tendency?* New Museum. https://www.newmuseum.org/blog/view/para-sites-like-us-what-is-this-para-sitic-tendency

Greer, S. (2004). *Four way bet: How devolution has led to four different models for the NHS.* The Constitution Unit. www.ucl.ac.uk/constitution-unit/

Greer, S. L. (2016). Devolution and health in the UK: Policy and its lessons since 1998. *British Medical Bulletin, 118*(1), 16–24. https://doi.org/10.1093/ bmb/ldw013

Gregory, R. G. (1980). Community arts and the need for openness. In B. Ross, S. Brown, & S. Kennedy (Eds.), *Community arts principles and practices* (Vol. 20). The Shelton Trust.

Griffiths, W. (2016). We love the NHS so much it is killing us. *Huffington Post.* https://www.huffingtonpost.co.uk/william-kloverod-griffiths/nhs-reform-future_b_13296520.html

Hall, S. (2001). *The multicultural question.* The Open University Press.

Haldane, D., & Loppert, S. (1999). *The arts in healthcare: Learning from experience.* The Kings Fund.

Hancock, M. (2018). The power of the arts and social activities to improve the nation's health. https://www.gov.uk/government/speeches/the-power-of-the-arts-and-social-activities-to-improve-the-nations-health

Hancock, M. (2020). The future of healthcare. Speech transcript downloaded from the Department of Health and Social Care. https://www.gov.uk/government/speeches/the-future-of-healthcare

Hare, G. (1991). John Guez: Busking, popular culture and cultural democracy. *French Cultural Studies, 2,* 153–163.

Harrop, A. & Phibbs, T. (2017). Time to transform. In *Local and national. How the public wants the NHS to be both* (pp. 4–5). The Fabian Society.

Hart, J. T. (1988). *A new kind of doctor: The general practitioners part in the health of the community.* Merlin Press.

Harvie, J. (2013). *Fair play: Art, performance and neoliberalism.* Palgrave McMillan.

Hayek, F. (1944). *The road to serfdom.* Chicago University Press.

Hayek, F. (1960). *The constitution of liberty.* University of Chicago Press.

Heath, I. (2007). In defence of a national sickness service. *BMJ (Clinical Research Edition), 334*(7583), 19. https://doi.org/10.1136/bmj.39066.541678.B7

Hebron, D. (2018). What I have learned from my time at LAHF. Blog downloadedhttps://lahf.wordpress.com/2018/10/01/what-i-have-learned-in-my-time-at-lahf/

Hechter, M. (1975). *Internal colonialism: The Celtic fringe in British national development, 1536–1966.* University of California Press.

Hepworth, B. (1970). *A pictorial autobiography* (p. 50). Tate Publishing. https://www.studiointernational.com/index.php/barbara-hepworth-the-hospital-drawings

Heseltine, M. (1981). It took a riot: The problems of Merseyside, the Toxteth riots. [declassified 2011]. https://www.margaretthatcher.org/document/127058

Hicks, D. (2021). The museum must change. https://www.aljazeera.com/features/2021/2/3/the-museum-must-change-a-qa-with-dan-hicks

Higgins, A. (2016). *Positioning arts, culture and heritage within Oldham council's public health priorities.* Local Government Association blog: https://www.local.gov.uk/case-studies/positioning-arts-culture-and-heritage-within-oldham-councils-public-health-priorities

Higgins, C. (2017). Phil Collins: Why I took a Soviet statue of Engels across Europe to Manchester. *The Guardian.* https://www.theguardian.com/

artanddesign/2017/jun/30/phil-collins-why-i-took-a-soviet-statue-of-engels-across-europe-to-manchester

Hill, A. (1948). *Art versus illness, a story of art therapy*. Allen and Unwin.

Hillier, B., & Hanson, J. (1984). *The social logic of space*. Cambridge University Press.

Hodgson, H. (1963). Medical ethics and controlled trials [letter]. *British Medical Journal, 5431*(1963), 1339–1340.

Hogan, S. (2001). *Healing arts: The history of art therapy*. Jessica Kingsley Publishers.

Holden, J., Kieffer, J., Newbiggin, L., & Wright, S. (2014). Towards plan B: A different approach to public funding of the arts. https://www.a-n.co.uk/news/towards-plan-b-a-different-approach-to-arts-funding/

Hooks, B. (1981). *Aint i a woman: Black women and feminism*. Pluto Classics.

Hope, S. (2011). Participating in the 'wrong' way? Practice based research into cultural democracy and the commissioning of art to effect social change. Birkbeck. PhD, University of London.

Howarth, A. (2017). *Dancing to a different tune: The contribution of arts to health*. Haygarth Lecture, University of Chester. https://www.chester.ac.uk/node/41127

Howarth, A. (2020). Online launch of the National Centre for Creative Health. https://www.youtube.com/watch?v=o6DEHuDVCIA

Howarth, A. (2022). Hansard, Column 1216. Volume 817. The Health and Social Care Bill. https://hansard.parliament.uk/Lords/2022-01-13/debates/2FDA3C76-9231-4D5F-BFD7-8D54B3A99A20/HealthAndCareBill#contribution-2B806DA9-BFE9-44AB-BAB8-8C4CA9E44775

Hunt, J. (2015). Making healthcare more human centred and not system centred. https://www.gov.uk/government/speeches/making-healthcare-more-human-centred-and-not-system-centred

Illich, I. (1979). *Medical nemesis: The expropriation of health*. Bantam Books.

Ingram, R. (2020). *Retreat: How the counterculture invented wellness*. Repeater Books.

Jackson, J. (1984). Address before the Democratic National Convention. https://www.pbs.org/wgbh/pages/frontline/jesse/speeches/jesse84speech.html

Jeffers, A. (2017). *Introduction to culture, democracy and the right to make art: The British community arts movement* (pp. 1–32). Bloomsbury Collections.

Jeffers, A., & Moriarty, G. (2017). *Cultural democracy and the right to make art*. Bloomsbury Publishers.

Jeffries, S. (2021). *Everything, all the time, everywhere: How we became post-modern*. Verso.

Jenkins, S. (2021, July). The return of the celts: Why a reawakening of national identities could spell the end of the United Kingdom. *The New Statesman*. Retrieved from https://www.newstatesman.com/politics/2021/07/return-celts

Johnes, M. (2019). *Wales: England's colony? The conquest, assimilation and recreation of Wales*. Parthian Books.

Johnson, B. (2020). Boris Johnson Claims Devolution a disaster and blasts Holyrood as Blair's biggest mistake. https://www.dailyrecord.co.uk/news/politics/boris-johnson-claimed-devolution-been-23021035

Johnson, B. (2022). Prime Minister: "Levelling Up is our mission and we're getting on with the job of delivering it. https://www.gov.uk/government/news/prime-minister-levelling-up-is-our-mission-and-were-getting-on-with-the-job-of-delivering-it

Jolly, R. J. (2016). Fictions of the human right to health: Writing against the postcolonial exotic in western medicine. In S. Atkinson, J. McNaughton, & J. Richards (Eds.), *The Edinburgh companion to the critical medical humanities* (pp. 527–540). Edinburgh University Press. http://www.jstor.org/stable/10.3366/j.ctt1bgzddd.35

Jones, K. (2003). Geborgenheit in a paradise garden: The architecture of the Bromley-by-Bow Centre. https://www.academia.edu/2570488/Geborgenheit_in_a_Paradise_Garden_The_architecture_of_the_Bromley_by_Bow_Centre_A_LITERATURE_REVIEW_AND_CASE_STUDY

Jones, J. (2012). From sculpture to scalpel. Barbara Hepworth's surgical sketches. https://www.theguardian.com/artanddesign/2012/oct/24/barbara-hepworth-hospital-drawings

Jones, S. (2019). Artists' livelihoods: The artists in arts policy conundrum. Doctoral thesis (PhD), Manchester Metropolitan University.

Jones, C. (2022). *From despair to where? Can the future generations act create a sustainable Wales?* Regional Studies Association. Downloaded May 2022. https://regions.regionalstudies.org/ezine/article/issue-12-spotlight-sustainable-wales/

Joss, T. (2008b). New flow, a better future for artists, citizens and the state. Mission Models Money. https://www.culturehive.co.uk/wp-content/uploads/2020/10/23974669-New-Flow-A-Better-Future-for-Artists-Citizens-and-the-State-Tim-Joss-2008_0-1.pdf

Joss, T. (2014). Healthy evidence. https://www.artsprofessional.co.uk/magazine/273/feature/healthy-evidence

Joss, T. (2016). Arts in health conference & showcase for health. Aesop. https://ae-sop.org/conference-showcase/

Joss, T. (2018). Will the NHS count the cost if it doesn't harness healing power of the arts? The Stage. https://www.thestage.co.uk/features/will-the-nhs-countthe-cost-if-it-doesnt-harness-healing-power-of-the-arts

Judge, K., & Bauld, L. (2006). Learning from policy failure? Health action zones in England. *European Journal of Public Health, 16*(4), 341–343.

Kelly, O. (1984). *Community, art, and the state: Storming the citadels.* Comedia.

Kelly-Irving, M., Ball, W., Bambra, C. Delpierre, C. Dundas, R. Lynch, J. McCartney, G.& Smith, K (2022): Falling down the rabbit hole? Methodological, conceptual and policy issues in current health inequalities

research,   Critical   Public   Health,   https://doi.org/10.1080/0958159
6.2022.2036701
Kenyes, M. (1945). 'The Arts Council: Its Policy and Its Hopes', Annual Report.
The Arts Council of Great Britain, London: Arts Council of Great Britain, p. 21.
Kester, G. (2004). *Conversation pieces: Community and communication in modern
art.* University of California Press.
Kester, G. (2005). Conversation pieces: The role of dialogue in socially engaged
art. In Z. Kucor & S. Leung (Eds.), *Theory in contemporary art since 1985.*
Blackwell.
Kester, G. (2012). Introduction to Gallery as Community; art, education, politics.
Steedman, M., (ed). Whitechapel Gallery Ventures. pp. 6.
Kings Fund. (2021). Integrated care systems explained. Making sense of sys-
tems, places, neighbourhoods. https://www.kingsfund.org.uk/publications/
integrated-care-systems-explained
Kwon, M. (2002). *One place after another: Site specific art and locational identity.*
MIT Press.
Kynaston, D. (2008). *Austerity Britain, 1945–51. Tales of a New Jerusalem*
(pp. 64–65). Bloomsbury.
Land, J. (2018). Why neoliberals are pushing accountable care worldwide. *New
Internationalist.* https://newint.org/features/web-exclusive/2018/04/23/
neoliberal-institutions-accountable-care-organizations
Labour Party Manifesto. (2017). For the many not the few. https://labour.org.
uk/wp-content/uploads/2017/10/labour-manifesto-2017.pdf
Laylard, R. (2011). *Happiness: Lessons from a new Science.* Penguin.
Lee, J. (1965). *HM government: A policy for the arts.* The First Steps.
Leeson, L. (2017). *Art: Process: Change: Inside a socially situated practice.*
Routledge.
Leggett, M. (2012). Art and economics (documentation). https://www.
mikeleggett.com.au/projects/inn7o-–-art-economics-documentation/
Letwin, O. (1984). In records published as part of the National Archive released
in   2015.   https://www.theguardian.com/politics/2015/dec/30/oliver-
letwin-blocked-help-for-black-youth-after-1985-riots
Leyshon, A. (2021). Uneven development, 'left behind places' and 'levelling up'
in a time of crisis. *Progress in Human Geography, 45*(3), 1678.
Lister, J. (2017). *The sustainability and transformation plans: A critical assessment.*
Centre for Health and Public interest. https://chpi.org.uk/wp-content/
uploads/2017/01/The-Sustainability-and-Transformation-Plans-a-critical-
assessment-FINAL-WEB.pdf
Lister, J., Davies, J., & Wrigley, G. (2015). *NHS for sale: Myths, lies and deception.*
Merlin Press London.
Long, S. (2016). *Book review: Contentious politics by Charles Tilly and Sidney
Tarrow.* London School of Economics. https://blogs.lse.ac.uk/lsereviewof-

books/2016/01/05/book-review-contentious-politics-by-charles-tilly-and-sidney-tarrow/

Lorde, A. (2017). *The masters tools will never dismantle the master's house.* Penguin Classics.

Lynch, B. (2013). Whose cake is it anyway? A collaborative investigation into engagement and participation in 12 museums and galleries in the UK. The Paul Hamlyn Foundation. Available from: http://www.phf.org.uk/reader/whose-cake-anyway

Lynch, B., & Alberti, S. J. M. M. (2010). Legacies of prejudice: Racism, co-production and radical trust in the museum. *Museum Management and Curatorship, 25*(1), 13–35.

Marmot, M. (2010). *Fair society, healthy lives: The Marmot Review: Strategic review of health inequalities in England post-2010.* Institute of Health Equity.

Marmot, M. (2015). *The health gap: The challenge of an unequal world.* Bloomsbury.

Marmot, M. (2017). *Prioritising and developing further action on reducing the social gradient in health.* The Kings Fund. https://www.kingsfund.org.uk/audio-video/michael-marmot-reducing-social-gradient-health

Marmot, M., & Wilkinson, R. (1996). *Social determinants of health.* Oxford University Press.

Marmot, M., Allen, J., Goldblatt, P., Herd, E., & Morrison, J. (2020). *Build back fairer: The COVID-19 Marmot Review.* The Health Foundation. https://health.org.uk/publications/build-back-fairer-the-covid-19-marmot-review

Marstine, J. (Ed.). (2011). *The Routledge companion to museum ethics: Redefining ethics for the twenty-first century.* Routledge.

Matarasso, F. (1997). *Use or ornament? The social impact of participation in the arts.* Comedia.

Matarasso, F. (2019). *A restless art. How participation won and why it matters.* Calouste Gulbenkian Foundation. Retrieved from https://arestlessart.com/the-book/

Mawson, A. (2008). *The social entrepreneur: Making communities work.* Harper Collins.

May, T. (2017). Statement from the new Prime Minister. 31 July 2016. (Transcript of the speech, exactly as it was delivered). https://www.gov.uk/government/speeches/statement-from-the-new-prime-minister-theresa-may

McInroy, N. (2022). *Levelling-up falls way short of what is needed.* CLES. https://cles.org.uk/blog/levelling-up-paper-falls-way-short-of-what-is-needed/

McKeown, T. (1976). *The role of medicine: Dream, mirage, or nemesis?* Nuffield Provincial Hospitals Trust.

McNeilly, G. (1998). *Group analytic art therapy.* Jessica Kingsley Publishers.

Merli, P. (2002). Evaluating the social impact of participation in arts activities. A critical review of Francois Matarasso's use or ornament? *International Journal of Cultural Policy, 9*(3), 337–346.

Mirza, M. (2006). The arts as painkiller. In M. Mirza (Ed.), *Culture vultures: Is UK arts policy damaging the arts?* (pp. 20–37). Policy Exchange Limited.

Misselbrook, D. (2014). W is for wellbeing and the WHO definition of health. *The British Journal of General Practice: The Journal of the Royal College of General Practitioners, 64*(628), 582. https://doi.org/10.3399/bjgp14X682381

Mohan, S., & Harris, F. (2021). After the death of Captain Sir Tom Moore, what role should charity play in funding the NHS? https://more.bham.ac.uk/border-crossings/2021/07/03/after-the-death-of-captain-sir-tom-moore-what-role-should-charity-play-in-funding-the-nhs/

Mold, A. (2013). Repositioning the patient: Patient organizations, consumerism, and autonomy in Britain during the 1960s and 1970s. *Bulletin of the History of Medicine, 87*(2), 225–249.

Moriarty, G. (2017) "Community Arts – a Forty-Year Apprenticeship: A View from England." Culture, Democracy and the Right to Make Art: The British Community Arts Movement. London: Bloomsbury Methuen Drama. 65–82. Bloomsbury Collections.

Mörsch, C. (2011). Alliances for unlearning: On the possibility of future collaborations between gallery education and institutions of critique. *Afterall: A Journal of Art, Context and Enquiry, 26*, 5–13. https://doi.org/10.1086/659291

Morsch, C. (2011). Alliances for unlearning: On gallery education and institutions of critique. *Afterall: A Journal of Art, Context and Enquiry, 26*, 4–13.

Morton, T. (2006). Are you being served? *Frieze* (101). https://www.frieze.com/article/are-you-being-served

Naismith, N. (2019). *Artists practising well.* Robert Gordon University. [online]. Available from: https://doi.org/10.48526/rgu-wt-235847

Nandy, L. (2021). How labour will root a new foreign policy in the home front. *In prospect Magazine.* https://www.prospectmagazine.co.uk/politics/lisa-nandy-labour-foreign-policy-global-britain-brexit-china-russia

Napier, D. (1996). *Foreign bodies: Performance, art, and symbolic anthropology.* University of California Press.

Napier, D. (2020). *I heard it through the grapevine: On herd immunity and why it is important.* Somatosphere. http://somatosphere.net/forumpost/herd-immunity-covid19/

Napier, A. D., Ancarno, C., Butler, B., et al. (2015). Culture and health. *Lancet, 384*, 1607–1639. https://doi.org/10.1016/S0140-6736(14)61603-2

Navarro, V. (2009). What we mean by social determinants of health. *International Journal of Health Services, 39*(3), 423–441. https://doi.org/10.2190/HS.39.3.a

NHS England, Public Health England, Health Education England, Monitor, Care Quality Commission, NHS Trust Development Authority (2014) Five Year Forward View. http://www.england.nhs.uk/wp-content/uploads/2014/10/5yfv-web.pdf

O'Doherty, B. (1986). *Inside the white cube: The ideology of the gallery space.* University of California Press.

Olusoga, D. (2017). Empire 2.0 is dangerous nostalgia for something that never existed. *The Guardian.* https://www.theguardian.com/commentisfree/2017/mar/19/empire-20-is-dangerous-nostalgia-for-something-that-never-existed

Osborne, G. (2012). Speech to party conference. Birmingham. https://www.theguardian.com/politics/video/2012/oct/08/george-osborne-tory-conference-video

Osborne, G. (2015a). We are the builders. George Osborne's full speech to conservative conference. https://www.conservativehome.com/parliament/2015/10/georgeosbornes-speech-in-full.html

Osborne, G. (2015b). Speech to Conservative Party Conference. Manchester. https://conservativehome.com/2015/10/05/george-osbornes-speech-in-full

Owens, R. (2022). Not only settlers, but rulers. The Welsh and the British empire. *Planet Magazine, 244,* 66–72.

Panich, L., & Leys, C. (1997). *The end of parliamentary socialism, from new left to new labour.* Verso.

Panich, L., & Leys, C. (2001). *The end of parliamentary socialism: From new left to new labour.* Verso.

Parkinson, C. (2011). *Arts and health manifesto.* Manchester Metropolitan University. https://www.artshealthresources.org.uk/docs/arts-and-health-manifesto-part-1/

Parkinson, C. (2012a). Fur coat and no knickers' in arts professional. https://www.artsprofessional.co.uk/magazine/255/article/fur-coat-and-no-knickers

Parkinson, C. (2012b). *A manifesto for arts in health.* Manchester Metropolitan University. http://www.artsforhealth.org/manifesto/

Parkinson, C. (2015). Devolution: The arts and health a social movement. Retrieved from https://mcrmetropolis.uk/blog/devolution-the-arts-health-a-social-movement/

Parkinson, C., & White, M. (2013). Inequalities, the arts and public health: Towards an international conversation. *Arts and Health, 5*(3), 179.

Parr, H. (1998). Mental health, ethnography and the body. *Area, 30*(1), 28–37.

Parr, H. (2000). Interpreting the 'hidden social geographies' of mental health: Ethnographies of inclusion and exclusion in semi-institutional places. *Health and Place, 6*(3), 225–237.

Parr, H. (2017). Health and arts: Critical perspectives. In S. Clift & T. Stickley (Eds.), *Arts, health and wellbeing: A theoretical enquiry for practice.* Cambridge.

Paton, C. (1997). Necessary conditions for a socialist health service. *Health Care, 5*(3), 205–216. https://doi.org/10.1007/BF02678379

Percy-Smith, J. (2000). *Policy responses to social exclusion: Towards inclusion?* Mcgraw-Hill Education.

Philipp, R., Baum, M., Mawson, A., & Calman, K. (1998). *Beyond the millennium. A summary of the proceedings of the first Windsor conference.* The Nuffield Trust.

Philipp, R., et al. (2001). *A report for the period April 1998–June 2001, including proceedings of the Windsor II Conference in September 1999.* The Nuffield Trust. https://www.artshealthresources.org.uk/wp-content/uploads/2017/01/2002-Philipp-Windsor-Declaration-arts-health-and-well-being.pdf

Philips, A. (2011). Too careful: Contemporary art's public making. In A. Phillips & M. Miessen (Eds.), *Caring culture: Art, architecture and the politics of public health*(Vol. 1(1), pp. 35–56). Sternberg Press/SKOR. ISBN 978-1-9341-5-71-9.

Phillips, K. (2019). A constructive-critical response to Creative. Health: The arts for health and wellbeing by the All–Party Parliamentary Group on Arts, Health and Wellbeing. *International Journal of Art Therapy, 24*(1), 21–29.

Philo, C., & Parr, H. (2018). Staying with the trouble of institutions. *Area, 51*(2), 241–248. https://doi.org/10.1111/area.12531

Pickett, B. (1996). Foucault and the politics of resistance. *Polity, 28*(4), 445–466.

Pollack, A., & Roderick, P. (2021). Response to the NHSE/consultation: "Integrating care: Next steps to building strong and effective integrated care systems across England." Downloaded from https://allysonpollock.com/wp-content/uploads/2021/01/AP_2021_Pollock_ICSNextStepsConsultation.pdf

Pollock, A., Roderick, P., & Price, D. (2021). NHSE/1 Consultation. Integrating care, next steps to building strong and effective integrated care systems across England. A response by University of Newcastle. https://www.sochealth.co.uk/2021/01/09/nhse-i-consultation/

Powell, M. (1997). Socialism and the British national health service. *Health Care Analysis, 5*(3), 187–194. https://doi.org/10.1007/BF02678377

Preciada, P. (2020, December). When states fall, Artforum. Retrieved from https://www.artforum.com/print/202009/paul-b-preciado-84375

Price, A. (2016). *Wales: The first and last colony. Speeches and writings 2001–2018.* Lolfa Publishers.

Pritchard, S. (2017). Artwashing: The art of regeneration, social capital and anti-gentrification activism. PhD Thesis awarded by Northumbria university. https://northumbria-sunderland-cdt.northumbria.ac.uk/Student-Profiles/stephen-pritchard.html

Pritchard, S. (2020). The artwashing of gentrification and social cleansing. In P. Adey, J. Bowstead, & K. Brickell (Eds.), *The handbook of displacement* (pp. 179–198). Palgrave. https://www.palgrave.com/gp/book/97830 30471774

Puebla Fortier, J., & Coulter, A. (2021, July). Creative cross-sectoral collaboration: A conceptual framework of factors influencing partnerships for arts, health and wellbeing. Public Health, *196*, 146–149. https://doi.org/10.1016/j.puhe.2021.05.017

Quilter-Pinner, H., & Gorsky, M. (2017). *Devo-Then, Devo-Now: What can the history of the NHS tell us about localism and devolution in health and care?* IPPR. http://www.ippr.org/research/publication/devo-then-devo-now

Raunig, G. (2009). Instituent practices, fleeing, instituting, transforming. In G. Raunig & G. Ray (Eds.), *Art and contemporary critical practice: Reinventing institutional critique.* May Fly Books.

Ravetz, A., & Gregory, H. (2018). Black gold: Trustworthiness in artistic research (seen from the sidelines of arts and health). *Interdisciplinary Science Reviews, 3-4*(43), 348–371. ISSN 1743-2790.

Raw, A., Lewis, S., Russell, A., & Macnaughton, J. (2012). A hole in the heart: Confronting the drive for evidence-based impact research in arts and health. *Arts and Health, 4*(2), 97–108. https://doi.org/10.1080/1753301 5.2011.619991

Robcis, C. (2021). *Disalienation, politics, philosophy and radical politics in post-war France.* University of Chicago.

Rooke, A. (2011). Arts and mental health: Creative collisions and critical conversations. Arts and Humanities Research Council (AHRC). https://ahrc.ukri. org/documents/projects-programmes-and-initiatives/arts-and-mental-health-creative-collisions-and-critical-conversations/

Rose, R. (1982). *Understanding the United Kingdom. The territorial dimension in government.* Longman.

Rose, N. (1985). Unreasonable rights: Mental illness and the limits of law. *Journal of Law and Society, 12*(2), 199–215.

Rose, N. (1990). *Inventing our selves psychology, power and personhood.* Cambridge University Press.

Rose, N. (2007). *The politics of life itself: Biomedicine, power, and subjectivity in the twenty-first century.* Princeton.

Royal Society for Public Health Working Group on Arts, Health and Wellbeing. (2013). Arts, health and wellbeing beyond the millennium. How far have we come and where do we want to go? Retrieved from London: https://www.rsph. org.uk/resourceLibrary/arts-health-and-wellbeing-beyond-themillennium-how-far-have-we-come-and-where-do-we-want-to-go-.html

Salas, R. N. (2020). Lessons from the covid-19 pandemic provide a blueprint for the climate emergency. *BMJ, 370*, m3067.

Samson, J. (2021). Levelling-up: A story from Bromley-By-Bow. https://www. powertochange.org.uk/news/levelling-up-a-story-from-bromley-by-bow/

Sandell, R., & Nightingale, E. (2012). *Museums, equality and social justice.* Routledge.

Schofield, C., Sutcliffe-Braithwaite, F., & Waters, R. (2021). The privatisation of the struggle: Anti-racism in the age of enterprise. In A. Davies, B. Jackson & F. Sutcliffe-Braithwaite (Eds.), *The neoliberal age?* Britain Since the 1970s. University College London.

Schreier, H., & Berger, L. (1974, June 8). Letter: On medical imperialism. *Lancet, 1*(7867), 1161.

Schulman, S. (2013). *Gentrification of the mind: Witness to a lost imagination.* University of California Press.

Scott, J. (1991). In I. Grewal, C. Kaplan, & R. Weigman (Eds.), *The fantasy of feminist history. Next wave provocations.* Duke University Press.

Senior, P. (1993). *Helping to heal: The arts in healthcare.* Calouste Gulbenkian Foundation.

Senior, P., & Croall, P. (1993). *Helping to heal. The arts in health care.* Calouste Gulbenkian Foundation.

Senior, P., & Croall, J. (1995). *Helping to heal. The arts in health care.* Sheeran Lock Fine Arts Consultants.

Series, L. (2021). Places like home. Blog retrieved https://thesmallplaces.wordpress.com/2021/11/20/places-like-home/

Shaw, K., et al. (2022). *The case for culture, what northern culture needs to rebuild, rebalance and recover.* Northern Culture All Party Parliamentary Group. Northumbria University. https://northernculture.org.uk/wp-content/uploads/2022/01/NCAPPG-The-Case-for-Culture-Report.pdf

Shilliam, R. (2018). *Race and the undeserving poor, from abolition to Brexit.* Agenda Publishing.

Sholette, G. (2006). Mockstitutions. Chapter 7. In *Dark matter: Art and politics in the age of enterprise culture.* Pluto Press.

Simpson, J. (2021). Review of *Contagious communities: medicine, migration, and the NHS in post war Britain* (review no. 1928) https://doi.org/10.14296/RiH/2014/1928.

SLG. (2015). Making it together: An evaluative study of creative families an arts and mental health partnership between the South London Gallery and the Parental Mental Health Team. https://research.gold.ac.uk/17789/1/Creative_Families_Report_b_0.pdf

Smail, D. (1996). *How to survive without psychotherapy.* Constable and Company.

Smith, R. (2002). Spend (slightly) less on health and more on the arts. *BMJ (Clinical Research Edition), 325*(7378), 1432–1433.

Sontag, S. (1976). *Illness as metaphor & aids as its metaphor.* Penguin Classics.

Sontag, S. (1978). *Illness as metaphor: Farrar.* Straus and Giroux.

Spandler, H. (2020). Crafting psychiatric contention through single-panel cartoons. In S. M. Squier & I. M. Krüger-Fürhoff (Eds.), *PathoGraphics: Narrative, aesthetics, contention, community.* Pennsylvania State University Press. Chapter 7. Available from: https://www.ncbi.nlm.nih.gov/books/NBK558324/

Spandler, H., & Carr, S. (2021). A history of lesbian politics and the psy professions. *Feminism and Psychology, 31*(1), 119–139. https://doi.org/10.1177/0959353520969297

Stewart, J. (2017). The birth of the NHS: Why wasn't it local government? In H. Quilter-Pinner & M. Gorsky (Eds.), *Devo-Then, Devo-Now: What can the history of the NHS tell us about localism and devolution in health and care?* Institute of Public Research.

Stickley, T., & Clift, S. (Eds.). (2017). *Arts, health and wellbeing: A theoretical inquiry for practice.* Cambridge Scholars Publishing.

Studdert J. (2017). Building real people power. In *Local and national: How the pubic wants the NHS to be both.* Fabian Policy Report.

Taylor, S. (1939). A plan for British hospitals. *The Lancet, II,* 946–951.

Taylor, R. (1979). *Medicine out of control: The anatomy of a malignant technology.* Macmillan Books.

Thaler, R., Sunstein, C., & Balz, P. (2010). *Choice architecture.* Princeton University. https://doi.org/10.2139/ssrn.1583509

Thatcher, M. (1984, July 20). Speech to 1922 Committee ("the enemy within"). speaking notes. *The Times.*

Tilly, C. (1978). *From mobilization to revolution.* Penguin.

Tilly, C. (1999). From interactions to outcomes in social movements. In D. M. M. Giugni & C. Tilly (Eds.), *How social movements matter* (pp. 253–270). University of Minnesota Press.

Tilly, C. (2004). *Contention and democracy in Europe, 1650-2000.* Cambridge University Press.

Tilly, C., & Tarrow, S. (2015). *Contentious politics, 2nd revised and updated.* Oxford Press.

Timberg, S. (2015). *Culture crash: The killing of the creative class.* Yale University press.

Toffolutti, V., & Suhrcke, M. (2019, May). Does austerity really kill? *Economics and Human Biology, 33,* 211–223.

Turner, J., Hayward, R., Angel, K., Fulford, B., Hall, J., Millard, C., & Thomson, M. (2015, October). The history of mental health services in modern England: Practitioner memories and the direction of future research. *Medical History, 59*(4), 599–624.

Underman, K., & Sweet, P. (2021). Counter-clinical spaces, sociological forum. Downloaded: https://onlinelibrary.wiley.com/doi/10.1111/socf.12783

Vize, R. (2015). The big devolution deal—or no deal? *The British Medical Journal, 19,* 360. Downloaded from http://www.bmj.com/ on 14 December 2018

Wainwright, J., & Mckeown, M. (2019). Place and race: Sanctuary, asylum and community belonging. In *Inside out, outside in: Transforming mental health practices.* PCCS Books.

Waller, D. (1991). *Becoming a profession: The history of art therapy in Britain 1940–82.* Routledge.

Walshaw, T. (2017). Art is not a luxury. Downloaded May 2022. https://www.paintingsinhospitals.org.uk/blogs/blog/art-is-not-a-luxury

Ward, K., & England, K. (2007). Introduction: Reading neoliberalization. In K. England & K. Ward (Eds.), *Neoliberalization* (pp. 1–22). Blackwell.

White, M. (2009). *Arts development in community health: A social tonic.* Oxford Radcliffe.

White, M. (2013). Acting local, thinking global in arts and health. https://www.communitydance.org.uk/DB/animated-library/acting-local-thinking-global-in-arts-and-health?ed=29971

White, M. (2014). *Asking the way. Directions and misdirections in arts in health.* IXIA. https://www.artshealthresources.org.uk/docs/asking-the-way-directions-and-misdirections-in-arts-and-health/

White, M., & Robson, M. (2011). Finding sustainability: University-community collaborations focused on the development and research of arts in health. *Gateways: International Journal of Community Research and Engagement., 4*, 48–64.

WHO. (1948). *Basic Documents* (49th ed.). World Health Organisation. https://apps.who.int/gb/bd/pdf_files/BD_49th-en.pdf#page=1

Wickham-Jones, M. (2021). Neoliberalism and the labour party. In A. Davies, B. Jackson, & F. Sutcliffe-Braithwaite (Eds.), *The neoliberal age? Britain since the 1970s.* University College London.

Wilkinson, R. (1996). *Unhealthy societies: The afflictions of inequality.* Routledge.

Wilkinson, R., & Marmot, M. (Eds.). (1999). *The social determinants of health.* Oxford University Press.

Wilkinson, R. D., & Pickett, K. (2009). *The spirit level: Why more equal societies almost always do better.* Allen Lane/Penguin Group UK; Bloomsbury Publishing.

Williams, R. (1959). Culture is ordinary [1958]. In *Resources of hope: Culture, democracy, socialism* (pp. 3–14). Verso.

Williams, R. (1962). *The long road to revolution.* Penguin.

Williams, R. (1968). Lost opportunity. In *Cultural policy collective, 2004. Beyond social inclusion. towards cultural democracy.* Cultural Policy Collective.

Williams, R. (1972). Cited in the cultural policy collective 2004 (p. 16).

Williams, G. (1979). *When was Wales? A history of the Welsh.* A BBC Wales Annual Radio Lecture. https://www.gwynalfwilliams.co.uk/when-was-wales.php

Williams, R. (1989). Culture is ordinary [1958]. In *Resources of hope: Culture, democracy, socialism* (pp. 3–14). Verso.

Williams, I. (2015). *Graphic medicine manifesto.* Penn State University Press.

Williams, F. (2019a). In a creative healthy place? Situating arts and health within the discourse of 'the devolution revolution'. Doctoral thesis (PhD), Manchester Metropolitan University. https://e-space.mmu.ac.uk/626298/

Williams, F. (2019b). *Facing inwards and outwards: challenging inequalities within Greater Manchester.* Manchester Institute of Arts, Health and Social Change. https://www.miahsc.com/news-2/2019/5/22/facing-inwards-and-outwards-challenging-inequalities-within-greater-manchester

Williams, F. (2020a). *Tommies, a very British haunt?* In a series, The Hospital Multiple. Somatosphere. http://somatosphere.net/2020/tommies-british-hospital.html/

Williams, F., Shaw, B., & Schrag, A. (2022). Enstranglements: Performing within, and exiting from, the arts-in-health "setting". *Frontiers in Psychology, 12,* 6291. https://www.frontiersin.org/articles/10.3389/fpsyg.2021.732957/full

Yoeli, H., Macnaughton, J., McLusky, S., & Robson, M. J. (2020). Arts as treatment? Innovation and resistance within an emerging movement. *Nordic Journal of Arts, Culture and Health, 2*(2-2020), 91–106.

Zook, J. (2022). The spatial dimension of hospital life. In J. Zook & K. Sailer (Eds.), *The covert life of the hospital.* University College London Press.

Index[1]

[1] Note: Page numbers followed by 'n' refer to notes.

149